# AT RISK

# AT RISK

## A JOURNEY WITH ALCOHOL ABUSE AND KORSAKOFF'S SYNDROME

**KARL MULLER**

*atmosphere press*

Published by Atmosphere Press

Cover design by Dhiraj Navlakhe



Keywords: alcohol abuse; Wernicke-Korsakoff's Syndrome; thiamine deficiency; addiction treatment; trauma; dementia

Atmospherepress.com

*This book is dedicated to:*

The doctors, nurses, and supporting professionals who care for patients and their loved ones who anxiously seek their guidance when facing alcoholism and dementia in all their forms.

The Alzheimer's Association and other dementia and neurological disorders organizations for their vital role in providing resources to families during stressful times.

Addiction treatment counselors and their organizations that offer hope and pathways to recovery.

Family law attorneys, supporting financial professionals, and family law court magistrates and judges, who compassionately help spouses, partners, and families with legal needs during already traumatic times.

Caregivers who go above and beyond to help their loved ones through their challenges of alcohol abuse and cognitive impairment.

Beth, my sister, who supported me and with whom we effortlessly coordinated care for Mom in her last ten years.

My therapists, Colleen, Katherine, Stan, and Dr. Marc, who helped me cope with my depression and the challenges of living with an alcoholic.

Co-workers, friends, and my family, who supported me during our difficulties and in my on-going recovery.

Kate, my loving partner, for her support and encouragement while bringing this book to life.

*The author is donating his net proceeds from sales of this book to the Alzheimer's Association and Alcoholics Anonymous.*

# Contents

"Man plans, God laughs."

*— old Yiddish adage based on the Old Testament of the Bible, Proverbs 19:21*

# Preface

## The Little-known Link between Alcohol Abuse and Wernicke-Korsakoff's Syndrome

Please sign here, Karl," said Joe as he pointed to the signature box on my bill-of-sale for my low-mileage, silver 2014 BMW 3 Series 320i. I needed a car. Since moving to Florida, I first rented a car and then used a friend's Chevy Malibu for a few weeks. It was time to obtain my own wheels, and I sat in Joe's office at the BMW dealership just off I-275 in Tampa. I once owned a high-mileage BMW 3 Series 320 in the early 1980's when I worked in France. I loved that car for its solid build and German technology.

After test-driving the car, Joe and I quickly aligned on the sales price, and we were now completing the transaction. While arranging financing and all the other details, he asked me why I had moved.

"Karl, this is quite a change for you, isn't it, from New England to Florida?"

Rather than offer Joe a vapid answer, I decided to be honest. "I'm restarting my life and am now legally separated from my wife. She is an alcoholic and became impaired by Korsakoff's Syndrome from her drinking. She's now living in an assisted living facility. "

Joe perked up. His head and shoulders lifted, and he looked directly at me. I had his full attention. He said, "I didn't know there was a link between alcoholism and memory loss. Can you tell me more?"

"Yes, there is a link, and I know more about both than I ever wanted to know."

Our car transaction was now momentarily on hold. He pushed

aside our papers, and Joe was intent on this conversation. I explained what I had discovered during my journey with Nancy. After informing him that I was not a doctor or medical professional, I told him I had learned about the connection between thiamine (Vitamin B1) suppression from long-term alcohol consumption and the resulting memory loss.

The condition was called Wernicke-Korsakoff's Syndrome (WKS). I told him my primary care physician in the Northeast – who had done his residency in downtown Boston – was well acquainted with WKS because it is often associated with poor nutrition and alcoholism. But Wernicke-Korsakoff's Syndrome occurs throughout society, and it is underdiagnosed. My doctor told me about an anonymous male patient who had been a successful, high-net-worth businessperson. He developed Korsakoff's through his habit of drinking a pint or more of whiskey every day. Sadly, this male patient was now living in an assisted living facility.

"Patients with Korsakoff's, unlike others with Alzheimer's Disease or other dementias, have the potential to restore memory loss if the patient abstains and has Vitamin B1 therapy," I added.

Joe's eyes shifted to a distant gaze just over my right shoulder, as if someone had just entered his office behind me. By the look on his face, I could see he was reaching back to a memory. Something that had once been puzzling to Joe was now clear.

In a quiet voice, Joe said, "I now understand something that may have happened with my wife." He told me *his* story. Joe's wife had been an alcoholic and became forgetful.

He said, "What you just told me helps me make sense of what might have happened to her. A few years ago, she decided to stop drinking, and over time her memory issues diminished." At the time of his telling, he noted that she remained a teetotaler, and "now I understand one possible reason why her memory problems slowly disappeared."[1]

Joe thanked me for sharing my story. We returned to the sales and financing papers, and we finished our transaction. The next day, I drove off in my BMW 320i and I had a new idea.

## An Information Gap

I decided that I could relate my experiences and supply resources to other spouses and caregivers about the link between alcohol abuse and alcohol-induced dementia like Wernicke-Korsakoff Syndrome. My conversation with Joe was not unique. During my final three years in New England and in my two years of living in Florida, I shared my story with friends, business associates, and even strangers on planes. Their reactions were identical to Joe's. Virtually no one I met was aware of the connection between alcoholism and memory impairment. Most people associated alcoholism with liver disease or diabetes, or they were aware of Alzheimer's Disease and other forms of memory loss and dementia. But *the link between alcohol and memory loss was not common knowledge.*

Some literature tells readers that WKS is relatively rare, but Korsakoff's is underdiagnosed.[2] A 2009 research publication concluded: "Reported prevalence rates [of WKS] at post-mortem are between 1 and 2% in the general population and 12 and 14% in the alcohol misusing population."[3] According to a 2019 NSDUH report[4], 14.5 million people ages twelve and older had Alcohol Use Disorder (AUD). This number included 9 million men and 5.5 million women. Out of an estimated 14.5 million people with AUD, up to 12-14 percent may be affected by Wernicke-Korsakoff's Syndrome (WKS).

In other words, over 1.7 million people in the US could be affected by WKS through alcohol abuse alone.

I hope this story, the lessons learned, and the resources will help readers support their loved ones who are at risk of developing Wernicke-Korsakoff's Syndrome or are already affected. Early interventions are important, and so is asking key questions of your medical, legal, and addiction treatment professionals. Answers to these questions could save years of diminished cognition and many dollars, and improve the quality of life for you, your loved one, and your family.

# Introduction

I wish this book had been available during my journey with an alcoholic spouse who later developed Wernicke-Korsakoff's Syndrome (which includes Wernicke's Encephalopathy and Korsakoff's Psychosis, often shortened to Korsakoff's Syndrome or WKS)[5,6]. I had no prior experience with alcohol abuse or dementia and knew nothing about the connection between alcohol and alcohol-related dementia. While substantial literature was then available about Alzheimer's Disease, vascular, Lewy Body, and other forms of dementia, I found few published resources for caregivers about alcoholism <u>and</u> Korsakoff's Syndrome when I needed guidance.

For spouses and partners of alcoholic loved ones who have or may develop Korsakoff's – you are not alone in your challenges and the need for resources. In this book, I share information about:

- Wernicke-Korsakoff's Syndrome (focusing on Korsakoff's Syndrome), symptoms, and the diagnosis process used in our situation.
- The unique challenges of placing my spouse, Nancy, in addiction treatment due to her WKS diagnosis and in obtaining proper care and support (including long-term care facilities).
- Questions you may wish to ask your medical, mental health, addiction treatment, and legal teams to discuss care for your loved one, including menopause when your loved one is female.
- Strategies and resources to help caregivers with their own self-care.
- Facing tough questions about loyalty, honesty, and codependency.
- Print and organizational resources you can tap.

While I am not a healthcare professional nor an addiction treatment counselor, I acquired significant knowledge about alcohol abuse and WKS. I bear the scars of living with an alcoholic and helping her in obtaining her diagnosis of WKS, treatments, and eventual placement in assisted living. You may glean ideas from our lessons-learned that you can use to enhance the care for your loved one for the diagnosis, treatment, and potential ***recovery*** from Korsakoff's.

You may be surprised – as was Joe, my BMW salesperson – to read the word "recovery." If your loved one has been diagnosed with Wernicke Encephalopathy and/or early-stage Korsakoff's Syndrome, some or all their cognitive function may return if they abstain from alcohol consumption and if they obtain thiamine therapy. But these efforts must begin early enough.

In this book, I describe my journey with Nancy, beginning with our first twenty years of marriage, and then her gradual slide into alcohol abuse, her diagnosis of Korsakoff's Syndrome, and attempts to help Nancy abstain. You will see the challenges of placing Nancy in long-term care, and along the way, you will see the difficulties facing spouses, partners, and families in coping with diagnosis, treatment, and care management. Of the most importance, you will see the impacts of critical information gaps that prolonged our journey, increased our costs, and added to our trauma.

When Nancy was diagnosed with WKS in 2012, I tapped the resources available to me at the time. While several books on dementia focused on Alzheimer's and more common forms of dementia and memory loss, limited information was available about Wernicke-Korsakoff's Syndrome. Moreover, I could not find any stories or advice from a caregiver's perspective to help me understand the combined conditions, how diagnoses are performed, what to expect in the disease progression, or the appropriate medical, mental health, addiction treatment, and legal professionals to seek out (besides the obvious, neurologists).

Nancy and I eventually found a caring team of neurological medical professionals, a private social worker, two addiction treatment centers, and a helpful state chapter of the Alzheimer's Association. Most friends stuck with us and supplied immeasurable support and understanding; some did not. My co-workers and my employer were understanding and gave me the time I needed to support Nancy and navigate our irregular path.

The personal trauma of living more than twenty years with Nancy's alcoholism and WKS led me to therapy, and later treatment for Post-Traumatic Stress Disorder (PTSD). My ordeal taught me important life lessons: *Be Grateful. Be Humble. Be Kind. Be Tolerant.*

When a demonic driver swerves in front of your car on the freeway or turnpike, or when a sales associate at your favorite store is curt or unhelpful, please consider that you have no idea what may have happened to him or her last night. Perhaps their child was diagnosed with leukemia, their spouse declared their marriage over and is moving out, or their father or mother passed away. Do others know of *your* pain? Probably not. A little patience and compassion go a long way in easing our respective burdens in life. I like to think that kindness begets kindness.

My hope is that this book will help you and your loved one better face the challenges of alcohol abuse and Wernicke-Korsakoff's Syndrome.

# Part 1

## Descent and Metamorphosis: 1970-2010

# Chapter 1

## The Early Years

Nancy and I were married for over 40 years. Our backgrounds were similar. We were both born and raised during the 1950s in Colorado. There and across America at that time, cities, towns, and the countryside were filled with returned World War Two veterans who were raising families. They were industrious tradesmen, farmers, shopkeepers, teachers, homemakers, salespeople, and many employed in the manufacturing sector who produced American-made autos and goods for the masses after WW2. These were members of the "Greatest Generation" who lived in towns and suburbs in row houses, bungalows, ranch-style houses, or Cape Cod tract housing built for them and their new families after V-E and V-J Days.

Nancy and I had been high school sweethearts who met through matcher-maker friends. We married in our early twenties. We were best friends, which is what kept us together through the highs and lows of a long, evolving marriage. We were devoted to each other in an independent kind of way. Together (and without children), Nancy and I enjoyed bicycling, rock climbing, sailing, hiking, and more. We were happy to do things together, but equally content to have some quiet time or a few days alone.

Our relationship appeared to be and was solid for the first twenty years of our married life. During the typical challenges that couples face in a long-time marriage, being best friends kept us together. Also, in our mid-thirties, we had an eight-month informal separation when I worked overseas in France. It was then that I realized I was suffocating in our relationship and needed time alone to grow.

After my return to the States, Nancy moved to New England where job prospects were better for her line of work. I followed her a year later when I also found interesting work there. It was a challenging time – new town, new job, and restarting our relationship. We worked on it and eventually bought a house. We had great neighbors, and we were both quite involved in our community.

That fulfilling life, which we had cultivated for over twenty years, gradually died. The slow demise did not occur because of an extramarital affair, a death, or through any of the usual reasons that two people cannot stay together. Our marriage ended because of alcohol abuse and resulting cognitive impairment.

# Chapter 2

# Slow Drift

## Gradual Descent

For our first 22 years together, Nancy was only a social drinker, mostly on weekends. Occasionally, she consumed a bit too much vodka during Friday happy hours, or perhaps one glass too many of a nice Sonoma County pinot noir wine at a neighborhood gathering. Sometimes so did I. Nancy's extended family had a history of alcoholism, but my family did not. Therefore, I was ill-equipped to either recognize or know how to respond to her growing alcohol excesses. My rationalizations of her increasing alcoholic behaviors did not help us either.

In 1993, Nancy's attraction to alcohol bloomed when she was 43 years old. After many years in a financial asset management consulting business in North America, Nancy embarked on a ten-year consulting gig in Latin America. She relished the work and the adventure of being overseas, meeting new people, and taking weekend excursions to historic cultural sites, jungles, mountains, and seashores. Nancy blossomed! She was in her element. Her confidence grew, she was intellectually stimulated, and her clients loved her.

While Nancy relished these amazing professional and personal opportunities, this time overseas also facilitated a personal disaster. During those ten years of foreign postings, she often spent three to six weeks at her assignment location, returned home for two to three weeks, and returned to her overseas work locations. Upon returning to her hotel from her clients' offices – *being alone* – she usually enjoyed two cocktails during happy hour, then consumed several glasses of wine at dinner, followed by a nightcap or two before retiring to bed. Every night. I saw this first-hand during a ten-day visit with Nancy during one of her postings, and she also told me of her routine. Her new pattern of increased alcohol consumption continued in both her overseas assignments and back home.

From my own observations of Nancy's drinking patterns, I compiled Figure 1 which illustrates Nancy's estimated alcohol consumption over a 43-year period. The chart ends in 2014, when she entered assisted living at age 64. Superimposed in this chart are limits of "moderate" drinking as defined by the National Institute of Alcohol Abuse and Alcoholism at 0.6 ounces of pure alcohol, standardized by type of beverage.[7] Moderate drinking has been defined as one drink per day for women and two drinks a day for men, as posted by the National Institute of Alcohol Abuse and Alcoholism.[8]

When her steady Latin American work ended, Nancy focused on developing new overseas assignments and refocusing on domestic projects. Her alcohol abuse not only continued unabated, it unfortunately increased.

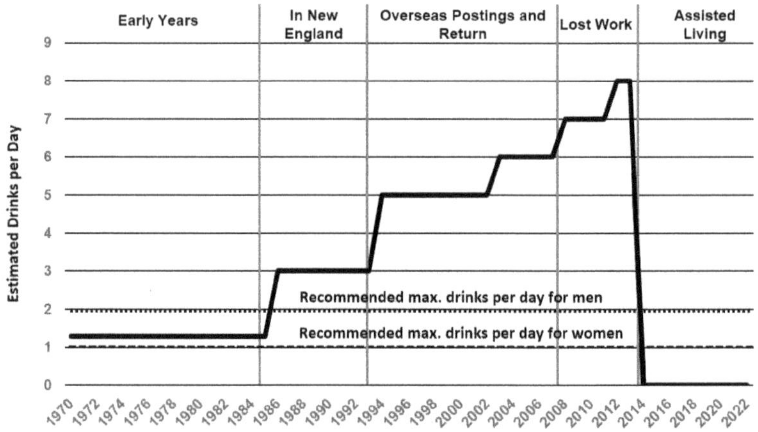


Figure 1. Nancy's estimated drinks per day

Source: Author

Towards the end, she consumed at least eight drinks a day.

I never understood Nancy's need for drinking. Why does someone self-medicate with alcohol? What triggered her alcoholism? Did she have an emerging psychological need that led to a new-found craving? Was there an underlying insecurity, self-doubt, or sense of unworthiness? Had I been unavailable emotionally? Had I been a bad husband? *What* was the trigger?

Nancy did not discuss with me the reasons for her increased alcohol consumption. In trying to understand the reasons behind the drinking, she either denied she had a problem or feigned concurrence with her need to reduce or stop her drinking, but she nonetheless continued.

After reading Kerry Egan's book *On Living*,[9] in which her work as a hospice chaplain highlighted the need to listen to dying patients, I could not help but wonder if more active listening might have altered the course of Nancy's alcoholism when I first noticed her increased drinking. Why didn't I simply ask her to tell me what was on her mind? I could have asked her more questions and *just listened – Why? What are you hiding from or want to forget? Are you unhappy?*

In *Never Enough: The Neuroscience and Experience of Addiction*,[10] Dr. Judith Grisel offers insights both from her own personal addiction experience along with her knowledge as a neuroscientist. I learned that consuming alcohol in moderate quantities reduces anxiety as well as activates pleasure and possibility. However, addiction not only occurs through the act of consuming but also from the *anticipation* of drinking (or consuming the drug of preference). Dr. Grisel notes that individuals with a family history of alcoholism are three to five times more likely to develop alcoholism.

Therein may lie the answers to Nancy's propensity to drink in excess. Her drinking may have been due to anxiety or some desire to forget some past events. During my journey with her, I came to learn about other potential triggers and contributors to her drinking.

# Chapter 3

## The New Reality

The frightening new reality of Nancy's alcohol abuse shook me one Friday evening in 2001 at my employer's annual year-end holiday party. Attendees enjoyed a four-course dinner, socialized, and danced in a swanky downtown hotel. However, as the evening entered its fourth hour, I returned from the restroom to see Nancy staggering glassy-eyed on the dance floor in her black cocktail dress. I swiftly intervened as quietly as possible, whisked her out of sight, and returned us to our hotel room.

Upon entering our room, I asked Nancy, "How can you embarrass us this way in front of my boss and my co-workers?" Because she was incoherent, that question was lost in her unfocused blue eyes and alcohol-muddled brain. In the morning, she had no recollection of the previous evening's fiasco.

In another instance in 2003, I accompanied Nancy to a business dinner meeting. She had been imbibing all evening, and as she participated in discussions after dinner, the effects were now painfully clear to all attendees. I soon became the target of several attendees who shot quick, furtive glances my way – *"Can't you do something?"* I discreetly returned these glances: *"Yeah, like I can control this?"* Mercifully, one of the group's board members soon found a convenient, low-key segue to end the discussion. After the meeting adjourned, several attendees took me aside in the parking lot and said, "I sure hope you're not going to let her drive home alone," with a mixture of sadness, pity (for her and me), and firm resolve that she was a threat to herself and society in her current state. I drove us home in my car in icy silence. We retrieved her car the next morning while running other errands, and she said, "Karl, why are we stopping at the restaurant? Was there a problem with my car?" She did not understand why we left her car in the inn's parking lot.

Over time, her drinking increased. Upon returning home from business travel, sometimes as early as 3:00 PM, I entered the house to find Nancy slumped over in my favorite easy chair. It occupied the sunlit corner of our cozy family room by our fireplace, surrounded by art, ceramics, and books from our travels. This nook was our space to relax. It became Nancy's drinking corner.

As her alcohol abuse worsened, I usually cooked dinner. I loved cooking, and it was (and still is) a creative outlet for me. I relished preparing restaurant-quality meals, but during this time, my appetite quickly faded upon seeing Nancy staggering to our kitchen table. In January 2013, a little over a year before she was finally placed in an assisted living facility, her drinking sometimes reduced her capability to even eat properly with utensils.

## The Good Old Days

During our first twenty years, our days were simple. Beginning when we were both 31 years old, we would wake at 4:20 AM, don our workout gear, and arrive at our fitness center when doors opened at 5:00 AM. This was our daily routine, except on Sundays when I would often jog in the neighborhood and nearby city parks. Our daily morning routines included strength/weight-bearing exercises or cardiovascular workouts. These daily workouts enabled me to maintain my weight, even with extensive business travel and its resulting uneven eating patterns.

When we were both working in downtown offices, we would change clothes and commute to work, usually eating separate breakfasts on the fly. After we both began working remotely, we would return home from our fitness center to prepare breakfast. We began our respective workdays in our third bedroom at our respective desks. Nancy and I usually ate lunch together on our large backyard deck or in the kitchen. Sometimes, I embarked on an extra two-mile run and would then eat a sandwich and fruit at my desk.

Nancy had more scheduling flexibility in her daily routine and was more able to better accommodate daytime errands. These efforts kept the household running smoothly, leaving us with weekend time for socializing and home maintenance.

Dinner preparation sometimes included a glass of wine or a cocktail, and we occasionally had a glass of wine at dinner – but not every night and usually only on the weekends. After dishes and prep for the morning, we were normally in bed by 8:30 PM, so we would be well rested for the 4:20 AM wake-up alarm.

As Nancy's alcoholism progressed, this routine shifted. Beginning in 2008 at the age of 58, she lost bids on new consulting projects and eventually lost *all* her consulting work. Word of her performance issues circulated within her professional community. As her workload decreased, her drinking started earlier and earlier each day downstairs in the family room, out of my sight. Her five, six, or more drinks affected our evening routines. We had little time for meaningful conversation because she was incoherent. When we could talk, our conversations often lacked any real meaning or purpose.

Hosting dinners with friends became a nightmare. We gathered around our long dining table, gleefully enjoying multi- course meals. As the wine flowed and the evening wore on, Nancy would often wax eloquently about some local news or (for the umpteenth time) tell us again about the historic sites she had visited while working in Latin America. She dominated the table, often repeating stories.

But the worst was yet to come. After the meal and some cursory kitchen and table clean-up, she often migrated to the family room's easy chair and continued drinking with or without a remaining guest. I soon gracefully ended the evening and ushered our guests out the front door from the disintegrating evening. I then faced the daunting task of moving her to bed. Attempts to talk with her about going to bed often were met with glassy eyes. She would pass out in my easy chair. I could not move her. The chair would be her bed for a few hours before she would wake up and crawl upstairs into our bed.

This sequence became the new normal. The physical and emotional energy needed to orchestrate and host social events at the house gradually became too much for me. Social events became exhausting games of chess. My mind raced with calculations judging her mood, tracking her alcohol consumption along with her quantity of food consumption, how long we should remain at the dining table, and when to shut down the evening to prevent friends from witnessing her vodka- or wine- soaked state.

Finally, by the spring of 2009, I could no longer face the tasks of hosting any more holiday dinners, birthdays, or Saturday night deck parties with neighbors. Our socializing ended. We became socially isolated, except for our morning trips to the gym and seeing neighbors around the neighborhood.

# Chapter 4

# Interventions and New Troubling Signs

## A Holiday Intervention

In the summer of 2009, we traveled to Colorado's Front Range for a ten-day vacation, staying at a mountain cabin beside the Fall River. We had invited Nancy's best friend, Chris, and her husband, John, to join us for the second weekend (which was also the beginning of a three-day Labor Day holiday weekend). They planned an early getaway from work on Thursday for their three-hour drive to our rented cabin to beat the holiday traffic. We were planning to enjoy an early dinner at 5:30 PM to kick-off our four-day weekend together. But around 4:00 PM, a phone call from Chris interrupted our dinner preparation. While they left work early as planned, the holiday traffic was much worse than expected, and they estimated their new arrival time to be close to 7:00 PM.

With their 4:00 PM call, we halted further food preparation, poured a cocktail for each of us, and nibbled on a snack during our wait for their arrival. While I moderated my alcohol consumption during our dinner delay, Nancy did not.

When Chris and John arrived, we devoured an appetizer of locally smoked freshwater trout topped with cucumber and horseradish cream plus other snacks. Soon we served dinner consisting of Colorado-raised lamb chops, garlic mashed potatoes, sourdough bread, and Caesar salads paired with a hearty California zinfandel wine.

A year had passed since our last visit together. Our conversations were lively and continued well into the evening. By 10:00 PM, Nancy was glassy-eyed and had trouble focusing. Nancy was on the brink of falling out of her seat. We all noticed this with alarm, and Chris encouraged Nancy to go to her bed upstairs, which she did with difficulty.

Ninety minutes later, Nancy reappeared at the dinner table and had little recollection of the evening. Nancy began drinking again while we continued chatting. Soon, Chris said, "Well, it is late, and we had a long, stressful drive. Time for us to retire. Can we help you clean up?" Three of us jumped up to dispatch a perfunctory table clearing and rinsing dishes for morning dishwashing. Nancy remained seated and continued her drinking. Chris and John said good night and headed to their downstairs bedroom. My job was to steer an inebriated Nancy into the upstairs bedroom.

Rather than join Nancy upstairs, I slept on the living room sofa – alone. I did not sleep well that night. I relished this time with Chris and John and was saddened and furious with Nancy for her evening's performance.

Just before dawn – it was a short night for me – I rose from the sofa, brewed coffee, and enjoyed the quiet as the kitchen gradually filled with the summer's warm sunlight. Soon, Chris and John sauntered into the kitchen. Nancy's room was silent.

While preparing her morning cappuccino, Chris took advantage of Nancy's slumber to remark about Nancy's condition. Chris lamented, "She's getting worse. She almost fell out of the chair." Whereupon she offered, "We want to help her and you. Let me try to talk with her. She might listen to me, and maybe I can persuade her to go to AA or seek treatment."

We then quickly settled on a plan. John and I would drive into town, run some errands, and grab lunch while Chris would initiate her intervention with Nancy.

As Chris and I finished breakfast preparations, Nancy appeared in the kitchen, and we sat down for breakfast. We talked about the great dinner the night before and our plans for the day. But Nancy had little recollection of dinner or her narrow escape from tumbling from the chair.

After finishing breakfast together and performing our kitchen clean-up, John and I executed the first part of our plan. As we left the cabin to drive into town, we told Nancy and Chris, "We'll grab some lunch after our errands at the wine shop and grocery store."

John and I first stopped at a grocery store and wine shop for our evening meal. We then enjoyed local craft beer, burgers, and fries at a nearby pub. We wanted to give Chris ample time for her intervention with Nancy. As John and I devoured our pub grub and beer, Chris started her intervention back at the cabin.

Upon our return, Chris said Nancy was out for her afternoon walk, and she quickly related the essence of her intervention before Nancy's imminent return. She told Nancy that she cared deeply about her and that she had been observing that Nancy's drinking was increasing. Chris encouraged Nancy to seek help.

Nancy repeated her usual mantra: "Yes, I know I need to control my drinking. I'll do better." This was her oft-used rote response in interventions, and later when she participated in residential and

---

**EARLY SYMPTOMS**

My initial concern focused on Nancy's growing alcohol consumption and the consequences. I did not make a connection between apathy and dementia or cognitive impairment. In retrospect, Nancy's cognitive impairment may have started well before I recognized her change of gait and forgetfulness.

I have since learned that patients with dementia can exhibit apathy, and which may be an early but often unrecognized indication of cognitive impairment. Apathy can also be associated with depression, so apathy alone is not a dependable marker for cognitive impairment. In the parlance of scientific research, it is a "weak signal" that is easily missed.

In retrospect there were several signs of this apathy. "Whatever you want" was Nancy's frequent response to my questions about her preferences about meals, errands, watching a movie, or weekend plans. She offered little initiation in socializing or household planning, another sign of this apathy. I just thought she was consumed with her business, especially when the overseas work was over, and she was trying to build her domestic practice.

---

intensive outpatient addiction treatment.

I welcomed Chris' spontaneous intervention that holiday weekend. I hoped Chris' observations and her offer of assistance might persuade Nancy to seek help. Also, I hoped Nancy would realize that others saw what I saw, and she might take the need to change more seriously. However, Nancy did not make any effort to curtail her drinking after Chris' weekend intervention.

## An Ultimatum

On January 2, 2010, after our quiet New Year's celebration, I gave Nancy an ultimatum: either she reduced her drinking, or I would leave. She agreed to curtail it, and we formed a pact to eliminate alcohol from the household. We also agreed to only consume non-alcoholic beer and wine.[11]

That afternoon, I emptied *all* bottles of wine and spirits in the house: an unopened fifth of vodka, a partially filled bottle of Bermudian rum, and all the wine in our meager cellar. I poured out all the alcohol down the kitchen sink drain.

I later learned Nancy surreptitiously continued drinking while feigning abstinence in my presence.

In another of my later attempts to intervene, I told Nancy, "I want us to be happy. You are an attractive and accomplished woman and my best friend. We have enjoyed so many good times together, but I cannot continue to live this way and I am worried about you. Can we *please* work together? I will stop drinking too if you will. I want to be supportive."

Her head nodded as she said, "Yes, I will."

## Other Troubling Signs

During 2009 and 2010, I noticed several odd behaviors.[12] First, Nancy's walking gait began to change from a normal stride to a wider stance with short, choppy steps, almost half-steps. I later learned it is sometimes called Korsakoff's Gait, and this change in gait was clinically significant. It is an indicator of Korsakoff's, but I did not know then.

Second, Nancy grew more forgetful. For example, as she drove around town on our weekend errands, Nancy would sometimes ask me for directions, "What's the shortest way to the Stop and Shop [grocery store]?" She was also resentful when I corrected her missed turns, saying, "I know how to get there!" She also had a series of small fender-benders with our two cars.

Third, I overheard disturbing work-related telephone conversations in our third bedroom where we both kept home offices. When Nancy's project director asked Nancy why certain key project tasks were not yet completed, Nancy rationalized her failure to perform by saying, "Oh, I had problems with computer software" or "Our internet connection failed. You know how that goes. Not enough bandwidth."

A few days later, after Nancy did not complete the project tasks assigned to her, the prime contractor terminated Nancy's contract. This was Nancy's last contract in her working life.

Fourth, Nancy's ability to cook diminished because she was having difficulty following recipes. For example, Nancy made beef stew one night. When I noticed three missing ingredients, I asked her, "Just curious, but where are the potatoes, carrots, and peas?" By this time, I had been noticing a pattern of cooking mistakes, but I gave her the benefit of the doubt. She usually said, "Oh, we ran out of them" or "Oh, I must have forgotten them." After our meal of her *ersatz* beef stew, I looked in the refrigerator and pantry, and I found all three of the missing ingredients. This example may look petty – after all, it was *just* dinner, and who among us has not overlooked one or two ingredients in a recipe in our haste to eat? But Nancy exhibited a pattern of forgetfulness.

Fifth, Nancy displayed a behavior I later learned was called "confabulation." Cognitively impaired individuals with Korsakoff's Syndrome cannot recall a recent memory, but they answer a question anyway, and often the answers are not accurate. She either omitted information or added false information. For example, I would ask, "Did you call Frank [our contractor] to schedule his next visit?" She would reply, "Yes, I did. He's coming on Monday." When I later checked with Frank, I learned Nancy had not called him. Or the reverse occurred. With Korsakoff's Syndrome, it is not a conscious act.

Taken altogether, these five behaviors were unsettling, and were *so unlike* Nancy. I wondered, "Does Nancy have vascular dementia (as her mother did), Alzheimer's Disease, a brain tumor, multiple sclerosis, Parkinson's Disease, or some other neurological disorder?" These observations, and her alcohol abuse, added to my growing sense that we should seek medical and alcohol addiction treatment.

In early 2011, soon after her 61st birthday, we began our three-year journey to orchestrate Nancy's diagnosis, neurological care, and alcohol addiction treatment.

# Part 2

## Medical and Addiction Treatment: 2011-2013

# Chapter 5

# Initial Neurological Diagnosis

Nancy's five unsettling behaviors suggested more than alcohol was affecting her. Despite all the pain and the disruption her alcohol consumption caused in our lives, I felt the need to help her find the underlying reasons for these troubling new behaviors. Nancy had no family to help and no other means of aid, and it was clear to me that she was unable or unwilling to help herself. Perhaps our relationship had some elements of codependency, too.

## Seeking Neurological Care

As a first step in addressing her unsettling behavioral changes, I asked Nancy to obtain a referral to a neurologist from our primary care physician (PCP). While our PCP supplied the requested referral, Nancy would not or could not make the appointment. This was the start of a new phase in my life. Over a two-year period, I scheduled the first appointment with the referred neurologist and later appointments with our medical team (a second neurologist, two neuropsychologists, and a psychiatrist) and addiction treatment professionals.

The remainder of this chapter and subsequent chapters in Part 2 describe the progression of Nancy's medical and addiction treatment care – including initial diagnosis through follow-ups and new referrals. The following chronological descriptions may prepare my readers for the challenges of managing healthcare for your loved one and the emotional rollercoaster of diagnosis and treatment that accompany diagnosis and treatment.[13] Hopefully, these experiences will help you guide your interaction with healthcare and addiction treatment professionals.

## Our First Neurologist

We drove to a nearby, nondescript, suburban professional building for our first consultation with Dr. Smith, a neurologist in private practice with one other neurologist. After we were ushered into his office, I offered my observations about Nancy's cognitive impairment, my concerns about her alcoholism, and concerns about new behavioral changes which might indicate a possible serious neurological disorder like multiple sclerosis (MS), a tumor, or Parkinson's Disease. Out of the corner of my eye, I saw Nancy's steely glare and set jaw. She was not happy sitting in Dr. Smith's office nor with the observations I offered to Dr. Smith. She was itching to express her disagreement with my statements at the right time.

Upon hearing my concerns, Dr. Smith said he would likely write orders for blood workups, scans, and other tests. Then, turning his attention to Nancy, he asked her to repeat sets of words, letters, or numbers that he read. Lastly, he conducted a brief physical exam.

In conclusion, Dr. Smith agreed Nancy should be evaluated for potential neurological ailments, and he passed us written orders for various tests. After his office received the results, we would be contacted to schedule an appointment to review the test results. Thus ended our first consultation.

I was initially pleased that Dr. Smith had listened to our concerns about Nancy's condition and followed up with testing orders. In the next six weeks, we completed all of Nancy's ordered blood workups, scans, and other tests. As I had hoped, these tests would uncover if her condition was caused by tumors, Lou Gehrig's disease, multiple sclerosis, or other neurological disorders.

Soon after we completed his ordered tests, Dr. Smith's office called to schedule our consultation to review the results. A week later we returned to his office to hear the results:

> "Well, I have some good news and some concerns. Based on my review of the test results, I have ruled out various neurological disorders. Nancy is not afflicted with Lou Gehrig's disease, brain tumors, multiple sclerosis, Parkinson's Disease, or other serious neurological ailments. But she is suffering from *some* cognitive impairment, but it isn't really that serious, and I'm not too concerned. I'd like you to return in about six months, and let's check on her situation again."

He prescribed Vitamin B12 therapy in the form of injections and tablets, but he did not characterize her condition with any label or description beyond "some cognitive impairment." Also, Dr. Smith said nothing about her alcohol consumption, potential Wernicke Encephalopathy, Korsakoff's Syndrome, or alcohol-induced amnesia.

Dr. Smith's diagnosis of mild impairment fed Nancy's raging rationalizations. As we walked into the parking lot, she turned to me and smugly admonished me, "See, Karl, it's not as serious as you are making it out to be! I'm fine."

But I knew she was not fine. Her drinking continued with the accompanying disruption of our lives, she was unemployed, and her abnormal behaviors were still troubling. I was underwhelmed by both Dr. Smith's diagnostic approach and his failure to address her alcohol abuse. But I decided to see how his diagnosis process would evolve.

Six months later (and with no change in Nancy's alcohol abuse), we returned to Dr. Smith's office for the scheduled follow-up consultation. As we walked into his building and into his office, Nancy was alternatively scowling and wearing a smirk on her face. Based on Dr. Smith's earlier assessment, Nancy was cocksure she was fine. She said, "I don't know why you think we need to continue this. I'm fine and you're overblowing this. I'm doing this to satisfy you."

Once in his examination room, Dr. Smith administered another battery of simple memory tests to Nancy, and he conducted another quick physical exam. His conclusions mirrored those of his initial examination. Nancy turned to me with a quick glance and a tight

"*See, I told you so*" smile.

"Nancy has mild cognitive impairment. I'm prescribing Namenda® and continuing her B12 therapy because it might help," he advised.

With that statement, our session was over. He offered nothing further about the reasons he was prescribing Namenda® and the thiamine therapy, only that it might help Nancy's mild cognitive impairment. He said nothing about the possibilities of Wernicke Encephalopathy or Korsakoff's Syndrome, nor did he express any concern about her alcohol consumption.

I was dissatisfied with Dr. Smith's second consultation. I appreciated his first efforts to rule out various neurological disorders, but his dismissive attitude about the seriousness of her condition was unsettling. Moreover, he said nothing about her alcohol consumption. In retrospect, I should have asked Dr. Smith for more details about his diagnosis and treatment plan.

---

**TRUST YOUR INSTINCTS**

If you are a caregiver, I suggest that you remain vigilant about the quality of care provided to your loved one. Ask questions. If something does not seem right, do not hesitate to switch providers or at least to obtain a second opinion. Moreover, ask health care and addiction treatment providers if they have experience with patients with Wernicke-Korsakoff's Syndrome.

---

That evening, as I prepared dinner, my instincts told me I should seek a second opinion. Dr. Smith was too cavalier about Nancy's condition. The next morning, before I launched into my normal workday, I located a comprehensive multi-disciplinary neurological center within a well-respected hospital and clinic in our area. Chapter 6 describes our consultation with this neurological care unit where we obtained a complete diagnosis and path forward for us.

Months later, I learned that other dementia caregivers shared my concerns about Dr. Smith. One evening, I sat in a sparsely furnished, multi-purpose room in a local senior center with our monthly Dementia Support Group, sponsored by the state chapter of the Alzheimer's

Association. My fellow caregivers were mostly spouses of loved ones who were suffering from Alzheimer's, vascular, Lewy Body, frontal lobe, or other forms or combinations of dementia. I was the sole caregiver in the group whose loved one was diagnosed with Korsakoff's Syndrome.

During the regular roundtable segment, one member asked if anyone could recommend a neurologist. She was unhappy with her husband's current neurologist. To my surprise, she added, "Dr. Smith is too passive, and he's dismissive of my husband's condition." Two or three other support group members nodded their heads and chimed in, "Oh yes, we left his practice, too, for the same reasons. He minimized the condition of my husband, and we're so glad we left his practice and found another neurologist." I was stunned, as I realized that I had not been off the mark.

The moral of the story – trust your judgment, be vigilant about your healthcare providers, obtain second opinions, and be your loved one's advocate. If your loved one is an alcoholic and appears to be suffering from cognitive impairment, my experience suggests comprehensive neurological centers are better equipped to provide enhanced diagnostics for Wernicke-Korsakoff's Syndrome and alcohol-induced dementia.

# Chapter 6

# New Neurological Team

My internet search led me to a comprehensive neurological care center with neurologists and neuropsychologists. The contrast between their diagnostic approach versus our first neurologist could not have been more different. We did not return to Dr. Smith for any further follow-up.

## Our New Neurological Team

When I called the center to schedule an initial consultation, the intake nurse and I had a deep discussion about Nancy's condition and situation. He said the medical team would review Nancy's medical records (including the test results from Dr. Smith) and decide on the best approach for Nancy's diagnostic process at their center. He committed to contacting us within a few days with the name of our first doctor at their center with whom we would then schedule an appointment.

As promised, in the follow-up call from the intake nurse, we were given the name and contact information for Nancy's first appointment. The center's team directed us to Dr. Jones, a neuropsychologist who would conduct a day-long series of neuropsychological tests. Nancy's appointment was then scheduled for a Monday morning, two weeks out.

The required protocol stipulated that Nancy should arrive well-rested at the medical center for her day-long battery of tests. To facilitate those needs and to avoid any early morning traffic delays, we booked a room at a nearby business hotel to ensure our punctual arrival. We enjoyed a pleasant late-spring Sunday dinner on the hotel's terrace. With no conferences or major meetings, the hotel was blissfully quiet and the perfect setting for Nancy to obtain a good night's sleep.

The next morning, we arrived at the clinic at 8:30 AM. Promptly at 9:00 AM, Dr. Jones, our neuropsychologist, entered the waiting room, greeted us, and the three of us walked to his consultation room. For the first fifteen minutes, he met with us together. Dr. Jones was the consummate healthcare professional – kind, attentive, and carefully explained the day's testing plan. The morning's test battery would end at 12:00 PM, and I would then meet Nancy back in the clinic's waiting room. The two of us would proceed to lunch in the main hospital building, and return to the clinic building at 1:00 PM for the afternoon test battery. Nancy's testing would end at 4:00 PM.

Dr. Jones' assistant then led Nancy into the testing room, and I had ten minutes alone with Dr. Jones. He described the testing protocol in more detail and asked if I had any questions or concerns. As he responded to my question and observations, I felt heard as a caregiver and concerned spouse. I felt Nancy was well cared for. I knew we had made the right decision – this was the right clinic with the right multidisciplinary medical team, and we were likely on the right path for an enhanced diagnosis.

Buoyed by my hopeful discussion with Dr. Jones, I walked to one of the hospital's cafeterias where I spent a productive morning working. I then met Nancy promptly at 12:00 PM back in the clinic building as she appeared from the testing area. Under the noonday sun, we walked back to the cafeteria and enjoyed our lunch together, chatting about her morning's test. Promptly returning Nancy to Dr. Jones' clinic at 1:00 PM, her afternoon test sequence began. The bright, clear late spring day bolstered my spirits as I returned once again to work in the brightly lit cafeteria.

At 4:00 PM, Nancy entered the waiting room with Dr. Jones, who said his office would call us in about a month when the results had been analyzed. We would then schedule an appointment with him to receive the test results. Nancy was tired from the battery of tests, but she seemed in good spirits. We had taken a crucial step, and now we simply needed to wait.

## Results

Four weeks later, we received a call from Dr. Jones' office to schedule our appointment to learn Nancy's test results. On the appointed day, we sat in the waiting room, and Nancy was emotionless. I was fidgety with a mixture of hope and dread, and I was not disappointed.

Dr. Jones ushered us into his office. Nancy was quiet and stoic. Dr. Jones explained the test results and provided the bottom- line conclusion: "Based on these validated tests, I conclude Nancy has a condition called Korsakoff's Syndrome, stemming from excessive alcohol consumption."[14]

Nancy remained silent with her eyes focused on Dr. Jones. I gulped. Dr. Jones further described the testing protocols and how the test results enabled him to reach that conclusion. He then elaborated on the processes by which excessive alcohol consumption leads to severe thiamine (Vitamin B1) suppression, which in turn leads to brain damage and Korsakoff's Syndrome. He explained how memories are created in the brain and how these memories are recalled. We learned how the mechanism of Korsakoff's Syndrome interferes with those processes.[15]

Dr. Jones shared the unexpected yet hopeful prognosis: "Unlike other forms of dementia, if Nancy abstains and follows our thiamine therapy regime, some or all her cognitive function might be restored. Some patients' memory functions are almost fully restored, while others find partial restoration. In twenty-five percent of patients, no memory restoration occurs. In part, the extent of recovery depends on how early the diagnosis is made in the disease's progression."[16]

For any restoration, patients must stop drinking. Dr. Jones encouraged us to engage Nancy in formal addiction treatment, and his center would likely start Nancy on thiamine (Vitamin B1) therapy.

> **HOPE FOR REVERSAL**
>
> Cognitive impairment associated with Wernicke-Korsakoff's Syndrome may be reversible, if diagnosed early and thiamine therapy is administered and if your loved one abstains. This is one crucial difference between impairment associated with Korsakoff's versus Alzheimer's and other forms of dementia.

After the initial shock of the diagnosis, I was nonetheless buoyed with hope when Dr. Jones told us about the possibility of partial or total reversal. Nancy was silent, biting her lips, and held a defiant countenance.

In concluding the appointment, Dr. Jones explained we should now make an appointment to see Dr. Edwards, the center's head of neurology, and we should repeat the neuropsychological testing in a year to identify any changes in Nancy's cognitive impairment associated with Korsakoff's.

Dr. Jones then turned and focused his gaze on Nancy with a mixture of care and concern and said, "Nancy, you are still relatively young, and you have many years to enjoy life and your time together. I really hope you can find a way to stop drinking and get professional addiction treatment support to do so."

I recall little about our drive back home in the early afternoon traffic. Nancy was mostly silent, and I could not tell how or if she had absorbed the testing results. My mind raced as I began planning my search for an addiction treatment facility. Upon arriving home, Nancy declared, "I am not committing to enter alcohol addiction treatment."

## Next Stop: Our New Neurologist

A few weeks later, as the summer's heat and humidity were building in New England skies, we drove to the medical center for our appointment with Dr. Edwards, the center's head of neurology. We were seated in a softly lit, wood-trimmed consultation room. Our black, hard-backed chairs faced her desk with a large computer monitor. Dr. Edwards entered the room, introduced herself, and sat across from us with a rather serious countenance as she opened Nancy's file. My heart raced as I prepared myself for her diagnosis and news.

She quickly moved to her evaluation: "Nancy, I've reviewed your test results, including all the scans, blood workups, results from Dr. Smith, and the results of the neuropsychological tests administered by Dr. Jones. I'm sorry to say that these test results, taken all together, confirm that your cognitive impairment is consistent with the diagnosis of Korsakoff's Syndrome."

The finality of Dr. Edward's confirmation of Dr. Jones's earlier diagnosis was sobering. On the computer screen facing us, Dr. Edwards then showed us Nancy's recent brain scans. She clicked through electronic "slices" of Nancy's brain scan and pointed out damaged areas on each scan. The scene was straight out of a made-for-television forensic drama series, *only this was real.*

As she shifted to another set of images, "Now I will now show you 3D composite images of a normal brain compared to Nancy's brain." Using her cursor, she pointed out the surface of Nancy's brain. "You can see here a series of rather widely spaced ridges and valleys." Changing images, she said, "Now notice in this image of a normal brain how the surface is tightly packed." In stark contrast, the surface of Nancy's images looked like a miniature version of the mountains and valleys of the Appalachian Mountains. It was visually shocking.

These images reminded me of a series of anti-drug public service announcements (PSAs) broadcasted on network television in the mid-1980s. These ads were sponsored by the Partnership for a Drug-Free America. In the most memorable ad, a disembodied hand holds a fresh whole egg above a skillet on a kitchen range. The voiceover says, "This is your brain." Then the hand cracks the egg into the skillet. As the egg sizzles, the voice says, "And this is your brain on drugs."[17]

Leveraging the visual impact of the brain scan imagery, Dr. Edwards looked directly at Nancy and sternly advised, "Nancy, every drop of alcohol is poison to your brain," both admonishing her and encouraging her to abstain. She also wrote an order for thiamine therapy which would begin immediately.

She reminded us that the partial reversal of Nancy's cognitive impairment might be possible, but this potential reversal depended upon Nancy's abstinence. "If you continue drinking, you risk further cognitive decline and ultimately some form of dementia."

She then explained the chain of events in the body beginning with severe thiamine suppression from significant alcohol abuse leading to Korsakoff's, which reinforced Dr. Jones' initial assessment. Nancy was silent, barely nodding to confirm she heard the solemn information imparted by Dr. Edwards.

---

**A CAUTIONARY NOTE**

At the time of Nancy's diagnosis at the neurological center, she either did not want to stop drinking or was incapable of stopping. Based on my later learnings about Korsakoff's, I believe that, by the time we obtained Nancy's formal diagnosis, achieving abstinence was unlikely. Patients afflicted with Korsakoff's lack self-awareness of their memory challenges.

This fact calls into question why our neurological team recommended addiction treatment. Our team may have thought Nancy's progression of Korsakoff's was still early stage, so she could have achieved abstinence through addiction treatment.

---

Shifting to a softer tone and countenance, she added, "Nancy, you really do need to abstain from alcohol. You are still a relatively young and accomplished woman. The good news is that your impairment is unlike that of patients with Alzheimer's or Lewy Body or other forms of dementia. *You may* still have the chance to reverse some of this damage. I really hope you will take this to heart."

As she slowly closed Nancy's file folder, Dr. Edwards glanced at me and then back to Nancy and offered another personalized message. "Nancy, your husband, Karl, is obviously concerned about you, and he wants to help. Together you can do this, but *you* must want to do it, and I really hope you do. Please abstain, and let's see you in a year. We'll have Dr. Jones repeat his test battery, and I'll see you again. I wish you well."

I remember her words as if this happened yesterday. Dr. Edwards' conclusions and directions were clear. As we quietly walked back to the car, I thought to myself, *"I hope Dr. Edwards' messages and the images of the physical damage to her brain might be enough to persuade Nancy to stop."*

During our drive home, we were mostly silent as I negotiated early rush-hour traffic on the turnpike. Later at dinner, Nancy surprised me by reversing her earlier position on addiction treatment. She agreed to enter treatment, though her tone suggested a half-hearted commitment. I said I would be as helpful as I could to support her. That night I silently prayed Nancy was now motivated to stop drinking.

## Becoming Informed

After these sessions, I began to seek out additional information about Korsakoff's Syndrome. A popular book for caregivers at that time was *The 36-Hour Day*[18], written by Nancy Mace and Peter Rabins, which included two brief paragraphs about Korsakoff's. I also sought out information from the Alzheimer's Association (US), the Alzheimer's Society (UK), and other medical and caregiver associations. But detailed information about WKS was limited.

While not available to me at the time, newer books about dementia are available to families and caregivers. Gail Weatherill's 2020 book, *The Caregivers Guide to Dementia,*[19] provides excellent suggestions on dementia-patient management and caregiver needs, as does Thomas Harrison and Brent Forester's book, *The Complete Family Guide to Dementia.*[20] While both books have a paragraph or two about WKS, little detailed information addresses the unique care needs of both alcoholism and Korsakoff's.[21]

Recently I found a 2011 book that would have been useful to us, but for some reason, it did not appear in various internet search engines I used after Nancy's first neurological assessment. David Steele's book, *Blackout: A Look Inside Wernickes* is unique because he shares the *patient's* perspectives on alcohol abuse and WKS. He describes his own alcoholic path that led to Wernicke's Encephalopathy and later to Korsakoff's Syndrome. Readers will learn about the difficulties in achieving sobriety and the frightening effects of Wernicke's Encephalopathy and Korsakoff's Syndrome. He came close to dying from Wernicke's

Encephalopathy. This book offers useful insights into the challenges faced by both patients and loved ones.[22]

These last three would have been useful to me as a caregiver after Nancy's initial testing and evaluations. However, at the time, my resources were limited.

# Chapter 7

# Initial Addiction Treatment

With the sobering but hopeful diagnosis, placing Nancy in addiction treatment became the highest priority, along with receiving thiamine therapy.

The world of alcohol addiction treatment was unknown to me. I was at a loss when faced with the daunting task of finding a suitable addiction treatment facility. The neurological team did not offer any specific referrals or recommendations for an addiction treatment organization that had Korsakoff's experience. In my state of shock on hearing the diagnosis from Drs. Jones and Edwards, I did not ask either of them for recommendations.

Naively, I thought placing Nancy in treatment would be easy, but placement was neither simple nor easy. I should have asked Drs. Jones and Edwards for recommendations of addiction treatment centers qualified to treat patients with WKS.

This chapter summarizes our experiences in finding addiction treatment for Nancy which were complicated by Korsakoff's Syndrome. I provide readers with key questions to ask of potential addiction treatment organizations that address these complications.

## First Attempt to Place

The day following our appointment with Dr. Edwards, I launched an internet search for residential addiction treatment and outpatient centers within about a three-hour drive from our New England home. I found a residential treatment center that seemed ideal based on their internet website: good reputation, well-credentialed staff, and lovely grounds. I called their intake staff, explained Nancy's diagnosis and her immediate need for treatment, and emphasized Nancy's perilous situation. With Nancy's power of attorney in hand, I completed their online application and authorization to access Nancy's medical records.

Within two days, the Center's intake staff called me with their decision: "I'm sorry to inform you that Nancy cannot enter our program. We do not accept patients with Korsakoff's." End of story. They offered no referral to a facility that might accept her.

## Second Addiction Treatment Center

Disappointed but undeterred, I contacted the intake staff at another addiction treatment unit within a well-respected regional hospital and medical center. I explained Nancy's diagnosis and her need to abstain because of her Korsakoff's Syndrome diagnosis. While this center did not offer residential treatment, I completed their application and medical records access authorization for Nancy's admittance into their intensive outpatient treatment unit. The intake staff promised a prompt return call with a decision.

Within 48 hours, Intake called with their decision. "We cannot accept Nancy into our program for two reasons. She is diagnosed with Korsakoff's Syndrome, and Nancy is not suffering from delirium."

I implored them to reconsider, emphasizing her neurological team's admonition that she *must stop* drinking to save further cognitive decline. They still refused to accept her into their program. But before I hung up the phone, I *pleaded* with them one last time to reconsider, as I was desperate to find treatment for Nancy. In the end, my pleadings were unpersuasive, but at least they supplied a referral to another local addiction treatment center that might accept her.

## Third Addiction Treatment Center

Unlike the first two organizations, the third center quickly accepted Nancy after reviewing her medical records and her application. Their intake process was swift and problem-free. Within 48 hours of informing me of their acceptance of Nancy into their program, Nancy settled into her private bedroom in their well-appointed residential treatment group home. Trees and a pond surrounded the facility, which created a sense of serenity for residents and staff. The home and the setting supplied plenty of nooks for reflection during the patients' homework between the formal one-to-one and group sessions. Residents received help from highly qualified and experienced staff, who were approachable to both residents and families. Nancy and I liked the facility and staff, and I thought it might just work for Nancy. While residential treatment cost a breathtaking $35,000 per month, a sizable portion was covered by my health insurance. And so began Nancy's month of monitored abstinence and addiction treatment.

On four successive Sundays, I drove to the residential treatment facility for their weekly three-hour structured visitations. Family members were offered these opportunities to see their loved one and

---

**MISSED OPPORTUNITY AND LESSONS LEARNED**

I missed an important learning opportunity with the first addiction treatment center. I should have asked these four important questions:

1. Why will you not accept clients with Korsakoff's Syndrome?
2. What have been your center's past experiences treating alcoholics with Korsakoff's?
3. What is the industry's success rate in addiction treatment with those with Korsakoff's Syndrome?
4. If an alcoholic is already confabulating, does an addict have enough self-awareness to be capable of learning abstinence?

Answers to these four questions may have saved two years of addiction treatment expenses and time. If we had learned earlier that addiction treatment was ineffective with Korsakoff's patients, we could have placed Nancy earlier in assisted living with monitored abstinence. Earlier placement might have resulted in at least some memory recovery.

---

to speak with staff therapists to discuss their loved one's progress.

Hour One began at 10:00 AM. For the first 30 minutes, family members met alone with their loved one's lead therapist. During all four visits, Nancy's lead therapist told me: "Nancy is doing all she is supposed to do, and she is also being helpful to other residents who seemed to need peer-to-peer personal contact." But he cautioned, "The problem is that I'm not sure she is really engaged in her own healing, or understanding the gravity of her situation. She's going through all the motions." His observations were consistent with Korsakoff's diagnosis as was her lack of self-awareness which had been noted by our neurological team.

After 30 minutes, Nancy joined us. She smiled as the counselor described her compliance with their program, but she was tense and unsettled when he noted her challenges.

In Hour Two, Nancy and I took part in the weekly family/patient group-therapy session involving all current residents and their families. These sessions were eye-opening. Patients in residence and their families had experienced deep traumas from addiction's effects. Their stories were sad, tragic, and sometimes hopeful. Several residents were turning their lives around: you could see it in their eyes, their body language, their facial expressions, and the self-confident way they spoke. They were ready to leave. You could see their steely determination to overcome their demons, to fully reenter their lives with their loving families, and do their own challenging work to beat their addiction. They were inspirational.

These group sessions were emotional rollercoasters for me. I felt empathy towards the loving family members who were hopeful that their loved ones would turn their lives around when they left the group treatment home. I thought, *"Would Nancy be a success story, too?"*

In Hour Three, the families and residents enjoyed a Sunday brunch buffet created by their in-house professional chef. Brunch gave each family quiet alone time with their loved one. Sitting outside on the terrace, Nancy said she was happy there as she regaled me with tales of the week, how good she felt, and all she had done. I focused on being an engaged, supportive listener, nodding as she spoke to acknowledge her and recognize her accomplishments. But I was haunted by the Hour One observations of her lead therapist.

As Hour Three ended at 1:00 PM, all the family visitors were gently but firmly reminded that we needed to leave. Residents had a full afternoon with group therapy, journaling, yoga, and meditation. Also, one or two times each week, the residents visited a local Alcoholics Anonymous group. The center was introducing them to this support system that they could later tap into when they reentered their normal lives.

During my drive back home each Sunday, I reflected on Nancy's condition and progress and hoped for her success. These sessions were mentally exhausting. But the Sunday sessions gave me hope that Nancy might truly integrate the messages from therapy, personal healing, and the tools to encourage and support her abstinence. Most importantly, I hoped she would embrace the need to change – *if she could change.*

## Discharged with Qualifiers

On Tuesday following the fourth Sunday visit, Nancy's lead counselor called to tell me they were ready to discharge her with the caveat that she needed intensive outpatient treatment. I was a bit taken aback. I thought a four-week residential treatment regime was too short given her extended period of alcohol abuse and the effects of Korsakoff's Syndrome. However, at that moment I trusted their judgment and accepted their decision.

Two days later, I drove to the residential treatment center for Nancy's exit session and to bring her home. First, I met one-to-one with Nancy's lead counselor, who told me that he and the residential staff felt Nancy had made *some* progress in self-awareness. Nancy had been diligent in her journaling and took part in all the individual and group therapy sessions, including the off-site AA group, creative activities, yoga and meditation, and the other requisite elements of their treatment program. But, he added, she still needed support to remain abstinent.

Then Nancy joined us in this final check-out session. We were seated in a private therapy room resembling a comfortable sitting room with a sofa, stuffed chairs, and windows filled with sunlight and greenery. Nancy seemed a bit buoyed and nodded positively when the counselor recapped her thirty days. Nancy liked the center and staff, and she had befriended her fellow residents.

The counselor reminded Nancy that she would now transition to intensive outpatient treatment at their main clinic. Arrangements had already been made for her to start in four days. When Nancy left the room to retrieve her luggage from her room, her counselor repeated his concerns about Nancy's lack of internalization of her situation. He was not especially hopeful that Nancy could remain abstinent by herself.

In retrospect, I should have asked the counselor: *Why are you releasing Nancy now? If you are concerned about her lack of internalization of her situation, is she capable of abstaining on her own or in your intensive outpatient treatment program?* I did not ask these questions, but I later learned that answers to these questions might have saved us tens of thousands of dollars and considerable time.

Nancy and I had a chatty return drive home just before the onslaught of rush-hour traffic. We arrived back home in time for her to unpack and settle back into our house before dinner. I prepared a nice welcome-home meal, and we sipped non-alcoholic wine that night.[23] Nancy told me about the outpatient treatment plans. She also told me she needed to find a convenient Alcoholics Anonymous group that would fit her schedule.

## Transition to Intensive Outpatient Treatment

Four days later, Nancy formally entered the center's outpatient program requiring daily commuting drives to their separate outpatient clinic. Those trips consumed her days. She left home early to be in the front-end of morning rush-hour traffic. She ate breakfast at a roadside diner along the way to the clinic, attended her day-long sessions, and returned home about 6:30-7:00 PM to eat dinner that I prepared. These were long days, but she seemed both accepting of outpatient treatment and happy having structured days since her consulting work had ceased. I was hopeful that these sessions would help her move to abstinence. I also appreciated having a quiet house during the day without any drama.

**SELF-AWARENESS**

Nancy demonstrated either her lack of will to abstain or her inability to do so since she lacked the ability for self-awareness of her situation as outlined by her neurological team. Discuss your loved one's level of self-awareness with your neurological care team before embarking on conventional addiction treatment regimes.

## Trouble Ahead

Julia, Nancy's outpatient counselor, conducted regular weekly one-to-one calls with me to review Nancy's progress. But after her first few calls, I received disturbing news and concerns from Julia. Nancy was failing the regular drug tests.

Less than two weeks later, I received an unscheduled call from Julia. Her tone betrayed the seriousness of this call. I swallowed hard, sipped my suddenly tasteless coffee, and asked the reason for this unexpected call.

Julia said, "As I told you several weeks ago, Nancy says and does all the right things in our sessions and appears to be the model client, but she continues to fail the drug tests. She is still drinking and if she doesn't stop, we will be terminating Nancy from our program." She reiterated their reasoning, "We cannot continue to keep non-compliant people in the program. It consumes our time and resources, as well as your money and health insurance claims, with no meaningful result." She concluded by telling me she had also informed Nancy of this dictum, and the next move was Nancy's. She *must* stop drinking now, or her treatment at their center would end.

The message was clear. We were at yet another crossroads.

Upon returning from the center that evening, Nancy said nothing about her discussion with Julia. I then told her about the recent calls with Julia, and she swore she was not drinking.

*Could the drug tests be wrong?* One or two might be wrong, but consistent false positives? Unlikely. I looked for stashes of alcohol around the house during the next few days, but could not find any. She either hid them well or was drinking to or from treatment, or while running errands.

The bottom line: Neither addiction treatment nor guidance from Nancy's neurological team had changed her behavior. The depressing thought occurred to me that Nancy's WKS may have progressed to the point where she was incapable of abstinence. Residential treatment, and now the compassionate but firm outpatient treatment, were not influencing Nancy's penchant for the bottle. At least Nancy's behaviors were consistent. She presented a good show. She may have thought she was being compliant – but she was unwilling or unable to stop drinking. Julia's call unscheduled call was sobering. I was now face-to-face with the likelihood that Nancy would not stop drinking. But the worst was yet to come. It is good we cannot predict the future.

A week later, I received Julia's final call. As expected, she informed me, "Karl, I'm sorry to tell you we terminated Nancy from our outpatient program today. We just told Nancy, and now we are telling you. She cannot return. Today is her last day here."

Even with Julia's earlier warnings and the previous week's "last call," I was still emotionally unprepared. I realized I might have to accept the fact that Nancy may simply never voluntarily quit drinking. If she did not abstain, Nancy would have no chance of recovering any cognition. Moreover, her neurological team expressed concerns, following Nancy's initial neuropsychological assessments and neurological exams, that Nancy's remaining cognitive reserve could be spent and she would decline further.[24]

In the week following the treatment center termination, Nancy attended a local AA group. Upon her return from the second session she told me, "Karl, those people have problems. I can't really relate to their issues or the people. I'm not attending any more sessions." She stopped attending this AA group, and she did not pursue other AA groups to attend.

Without a controlled residential treatment settling, assisted living, or another monitored living situation – where alcohol was unavailable to her – and with no addiction treatment support, Nancy would likely continue her daily alcohol abuse. Our next steps were unclear.

## Al-Anon and the Future

In retrospect, I should have sought help from Al-Anon.[25] I should have taken part in one of their local support groups. Had I attended regular meetings, I would have obtained new insights and ideas for next steps for Nancy's treatment as well as understanding codependency.

# Chapter 8

## New Outpatient Treatment and a Dead-End

Desperate to find another treatment possibility, I soon discovered a second well-respected outpatient center. During my first discussion with their intake staff, I described Nancy's diagnosis with WKS, the serious nature of her prognosis if she did not abstain, and my desperation to help Nancy find a pathway to abstinence. After their initial reluctance – stemming from her history at the first outpatient treatment center *and* her Korsakoff's complication – this second intensive outpatient addiction treatment center eventually accepted Nancy because her situation was dire. This center seemed like our last hope, and I was grateful that they accepted Nancy.

Nancy took part in several weeks of addiction treatment. Sessions were similarly structured to those at Nancy's first outpatient clinic – a mixture of group and individual therapy sessions, in-house exercises, and homework. Initially, her treatment sessions were conducted all day every weekday, though later Nancy attended three days a week.

In periodic calls and occasional one-to-one in-person meetings, Nancy's assigned counselor, Megan, told me, "Nancy is compliant with all the tasks and activities of our program, but unfortunately she is failing the drug tests." She added, "We're not sure Nancy understands or accepts her situation. We'll try yet to work with her, but if she does not stop failing the drug tests, we will need to terminate her from our program."

When I asked Nancy about the drug test results and the calls I received from Megan, Nancy continued to deny drinking. Whether through confabulation or by knowingly lying to me, Nancy was not accepting responsibility.

Shortly thereafter, in an unscheduled call from Megan, I learned Nancy was told she would be terminated from the program if she continued to fail the drug tests. This was her final warning.

I received Megan's final call a week later. "Karl, today we had to terminate Nancy from our program because she is still drinking. As I told you a week ago, Nancy is compliant with our program in all other respects, but she is consistently failing the drug tests. She is acting the part, but she has not stopped drinking. She was told today she cannot return, and it is her last day with us."

While I was expecting this final call, my heart sank. Yet another attempt to help Nancy achieve abstinence had failed. Nancy had been telling me that she had stopped drinking alcohol, only drank non-alcoholic wine or beer, and feigned surprise that she failed the drug tests.

I did not know where to turn next. Without abstinence, her declining cognition would continue unabated.

# Chapter 9

# Medications

Concurrent with Nancy's addiction treatment, Nancy's doctors also prescribed several medications. In this short chapter, I describe the medications and the two Vitamin B therapies which were prescribed for her so that the reader understands what may be recommended by their health professionals.

## Vitamin B12 and B1 Therapies

Dr. Smith, Nancy's first neurologist, prescribed Vitamin B12 injections and oral supplements. He only said that this therapy would help Nancy's "*mild cognitive impairment*" [his words]. Later I learned this treatment is indicated for numerous conditions, including alcohol-induced amnesia.[26,27,28] But Dr. Smith did not tell us this treatment was indicated for alcoholism. Moreover, he had still not explicitly expressed any concern about her alcohol abuse, nor did he mention that Nancy was potentially at risk of Wernicke's Encephalopathy, Korsakoff's Psychosis, Wernicke-Korsakoff's Syndrome, or other alcohol-induced memory disorders. Vitamin B1 (thiamine) therapy is indicated for WKS, but Vitamin B12 is not indicated for WKS. I am still puzzled why Dr. Smith did not tell us of the need for Nancy to cease alcohol consumption to address her "mild cognitive impairment."

Nancy's second neurologist, Dr. Edwards, prescribed Vitamin B1 (thiamine) therapy, which is consistent with a diagnosis and treatment of WKS.

## Memantine/Namenda®

Dr. Smith, Nancy's first neurologist, also prescribed Namenda® (generic: memantine) which is used to treat moderate to severe Alzheimer's Disease. It does not cure Alzheimer's, but the drug may improve memory, awareness, and the ability to perform daily functions.[29] When I reviewed memantine's drug information sheet, I did not see a reference to its use for Wernicke-Korsakoff's Syndrome. I could only deduce that Dr. Smith prescribed it as an "off-label" use of this drug for mild cognitive impairment [his diagnosis]. In retrospect, I should have inquired more about his rationale for prescribing memantine.

---

**VITAMIN B1 AND B12 THERAPIES**

If your neurologist prescribes either Vitamin B1 or B12 therapies for your loved one, you may want to ask these four questions:

1. For what condition are you prescribing this therapy?
2. Is the patient BI or B12 deficient?
3. Are you addressing the patient's alcohol abuse in your Vitamin B1 or B12 therapies or other prescriptions?
4. Are you treating for Wernicke's Encephalopathy? Korsakoff's Syndrome?

The answers will provide you with insights about the nature of your neurologist's diagnosis and treatment plan, and your loved one's underlying conditions.

---

## Effectiveness of Medical Treatments

Nancy's neurologists at the neurological treatment center stopped prescribing memantine and B12. In their place, Dr. Edwards initiated Vitamin Bl therapy. Oddly, neither Dr. Smith nor Dr. Edwards told us about the questionable value of continuing Vitamin B therapies without abstinence. I had informed them of her continued drinking.

As we saw in the results from Nancy's successive neurological assessments, her cognitive impairment had not improved and was trending downward. These results were not surprising because 1) her continued alcohol abuse would make Vitamins Bl or B12 therapies ineffective; 2) recent medical research suggests that some patients are genetically predisposed to ineffective processing of dietary or supplemental thiamine; and/or, 3) her brain damage was probably too far advanced at this point.

## Medications to Assist Alcoholics with Recovery

Apart from memantine and Vitamins B1 and B12 therapies, the medical directors of both intensive alcohol treatment outpatient clinics prescribed two medications for Nancy to reduce the appeal of alcohol itself.

Antabuse® (generic: disulfiram) is formulated to help reduce an alcoholic's craving by discouraging consumption. If alcohol is consumed after taking Antabuse®, unpleasant side effects can occur, such as headaches, nausea, vomiting, and more. I seldom saw Nancy take this medication, but on one occasion I observed it. Later that day, she drank alcohol and became nauseous.

I suspect she did not regularly take the Antabuse®. We know from the two outpatient addiction treatment centers that she routinely failed their drug tests. I cannot imagine Nancy taking Antabuse® while she drank alcohol because she would then become nauseated or worse.

Addiction treatment medical staff also prescribed naltrexone, which helps alcoholics drink less alcohol because it reduces the desire to drink. If Nancy had been compliant in taking this medication, its

---

**PRESCRIPTIONS**

Apart from Vitamin B1 or B12 therapies, you may want to ask your medical team about other medications:

1. What conditions of your loved one are driving the needs for additional prescription medications?
2. What is the effectiveness of these Rx's for your loved one's specific conditions (including, non-compliance with abstinence)?
3. What are the reasons for prescribing any medications "off label"?
4. Are any of these medications intended to treat Wernicke's Encephalopathy or Korsakoff's Syndrome?

---

effectiveness would have been questionable because she continued drinking.

## Final Word

Readers will note a common theme in my descriptions of our interactions with our medical and addiction treatment professionals: *Ask questions to understand their rationales in prescribing medications and treatment regimes.* You may uncover incongruities in treatment with your loved one's condition and/or health history. Conversely, you and your teams may discover opportunities to enhance treatment.

# Chapter 10

## Understanding Korsakoff's and Building a Support Team

When Nancy was engaged in residential and outpatient addiction treatment, I focused on two other important needs: 1) expand my knowledge of Korsakoff's Syndrome, which would help me understand future diagnosis needs, medical and alcohol addiction treatment options, and the physiological and mental progression of the affliction if unchecked, and 2) locate day-to-day support for us.

### Resources

When we first learned of Nancy's initial neuropsychological assessment results, Dr. Jones suggested that we review information about Korsakoff's Syndrome on the Alzheimer's Association webpage, plus another handy print-out on the website of their sister organization in the United Kingdom, the Alzheimer's Society.[30] Also, I found the Family Caregivers Alliance[31] and the National Organization for Rare Disorders[32] offered useful descriptions of WKS. These publications were helpful as starting points.

In my enhanced search for resources, I wanted to learn more: How to best identify initial symptoms and progression of WKS? What are the diagnostic tools used by neurologic professionals? How to best approach alcohol addiction treatment with WKS patients?

I found some information about the many forms of dementia, such as *The 36-Hour Day*,[33] but few resources were relevant to the unique nature of WKS.

Beyond publications, I contacted the state chapter of the Alzheimer's

Association to ask about their resources. They assigned our case to Richard, one of their chapter's social workers, who soon contacted us to arrange for a house call with me and Nancy.

## Alzheimer's Association State Chapter

During the house call, Richard conducted an hour-long interview as part of a needs assessment. Upon completion, he concluded that Nancy and I would benefit from the state chapter's assistance. He connected us with a community-based dementia support group that held monthly meetings in our town.

The support group members were spouses, partners, or other family caregivers, who attended the sessions with their loved ones who were afflicted with one type of dementia or a combination. The monthly meetings began with a brief joint session of both caregivers/spouses and their loved ones – which sometimes included a guest speaker who provided an update on dementia care or the latest research scientific findings. We would then break out into two separate groups: caregivers in one group and their loved ones in the second group. Sessions were led by three to four volunteer facilitators – one or two for the caregivers' breakout, and two for the patient's breakout. Each facilitator had experience with dementia care and counseling.

Newcomers were warmly received, and we felt an instant connection with one another. We were unified in our need to help our loved ones and to be supported by those who were in similar situations. My fellow support group members were empathic, open, honest, and knowledgeable. As a caregiver, it is comforting to know you are not alone in trying to support your loved one's experience with dementia.

Our support group was targeted at loved ones with mild to moderate dementia. When a member's dementia progressed beyond moderate impairment, they were required to transition to another support group for more severely affected individuals if they wanted to continue in this program. Their last meetings with our dementia support group were hard for everyone. We all knew the sad reason they needed to leave our group.

I looked forward to these support sessions because everyone there understood the challenges and welcomed the support. Nancy and I regularly attended the group meeting until I left our house and area in April 2014.

## More Resources

I continued to search for books and medical journal articles that may be useful to caregivers. I included these in the Bibliography and Resources section of this book. More recently, I found two booklets about WKS that are targeted at families and caregivers. Each contains brief descriptions of symptoms, disease outcomes, and resources.[34,35] As you expand your searches for information and support resources, you will obtain important insights to equip you in understanding the links between thiamine suppression, Wernicke's Encephalopathy, alcohol abuse, and Korsakoff's Syndrome.

I encourage my readers to tap these resources sooner than later, even if they are living with and supporting an alcoholic without symptoms of Wernicke-Korsakoff's. The insights you receive may enable you to start interventions, care, and testing early enough in the illness' progression to stave off more serious cognitive impairment.

---

**RESOURCES**

The Bibliography and Resources section of this book contains lists of written and organizational resources. These lists are not exhaustive; please consider them as a starting point for you.

---

# Chapter 11

## Menopause, and Surgery: Alcohol Abuse and Dementia

While writing this book, my partner, Kate, and I discussed the effects of perimenopause and menopause in the context of a range of medical and mental health challenges not associated with alcohol abuse or dementia. Later, I wondered if menopause or surgery on women's reproductive organs might increase the risks of alcohol abuse or dementia. I soon learned that such research had indeed been undertaken.

Relevant medical research had been addressing the role of perimenopause and menopause in increasing women's risks of alcohol abuse and dementia, as well as the potential impacts of surgery. When I initiated my literature searches (such as those through Google Scholar), I found numerous studies looking at the effects of surgeries and the timing of menopause on anxiety and depression that could put women at greater risk of developing alcohol abuse. While these searches for relevant literature were far from comprehensive, the extent of research and knowledge was surprising and compelling. I cite here a few of the studies reported in medical research journals I discovered.

Nancy's menopausal history was not explicitly discussed with us by our medical, psychological, or addiction treatment teams. They did not directly discuss with us the potentially heightened risks of perimenopausal or menopausal women for depression and the potential risks of alcohol abuse and dementia risks. Perhaps they thought it was moot at that point, but I include this discussion here because it may be relevant to my readers' situations.

## Alcohol Abuse

Scientific medical journals and relevant health care organizations have noted greater risks of alcohol abuse in perimenopausal and menopausal women. These heightened risks of alcohol abuse are *indirect*; these risks result from anxiety and depression from hormonal changes.

I found numerous peer-reviewed medical research literature addressing these themes. For example, in a journal article by Clayton and Ninan, routine screening for women in perimenopause was recommended because a "careful assessment for depressive symptoms can help identify the presence of MDD [major depressive disorder] in the menopausal transition. Recognition of menopausal symptoms, with or without depression, is important given their potential impact on quality of life."[36]

In a 2021 journal article by Conde et al., the risks of cognitive impairment and dementia from menopause were discussed.[37] In a third article, research results in twenty-nine studies were reviewed and compared as part of a 2021 literature review project. The conclusions illustrated the potential impacts of hysterectomies and uterine fibroid removal surgery on depression, anxiety, and other effects.[38]

Nancy's menopause occurred about the same time as she was working overseas in her extended postings. It seems reasonable to assume that Nancy's underlying tendencies towards alcohol abuse *may* have been exacerbated by her perimenopausal and menopausal changes.

About nine months before the beginning of her foreign postings, Nancy had a procedure for the removal of a benign tumor and an associated unilateral oophorectomy (removal of an ovary).[39] This removal, along with her early-stage menopause, might have added to her triggers for alcohol abuse.

In other words, Nancy's risk factors for alcohol abuse may have been heightened by early menopause, ovary removal, and the other potential triggers noted in earlier chapters (such as family history).

## Dementia

While I did not conduct an exhaustive literature review of the potential increased dementia risks in women stemming from the timing of menopause and/or surgery on women's reproductive organs, I wanted to ascertain if these relationships had been studied. I found medical literature describing such studies of enhanced dementia risks unique to women.

For example, a 2022 study found enhanced risks of developing dementia with early menopause (though not specifically citing Wernicke-Korsakoff's). This study included over 150,000 women in the United Kingdom (with an average age of 60). It identified those who developed Alzheimer's Disease, vascular dementia, and other forms of dementia. Researchers concluded that "women who entered menopause around age 45 were 30% more likely to be diagnosed with dementia before age 65 compared with those whose periods ceased at 50 (the average age at which menstrual periods stop in American and British women)."[40]

A Brazilian research study results, reported in 2021, suggested that changes in estrogen levels in women may play a role in their enhanced risks of developing dementia,[41] though again Korsakoff's Syndrome was not explicated named.

Nancy's surgery for the benign tumor and an ovary removal - resulting in early-stage menopause and a reduction in estrogen levels - *might* have increased her risk of developing dementia. One important caution: I did not see studies investigating the association of such surgeries or menopausal timing on WKS.

## Anesthesia and Dementia

During our initial consultations with our neurological team, Nancy asked Drs. Smith and Edwards if her anesthesia experience with surgery could have contributed to her developing Wernicke-Korsakoff's Syndrome. Her team said that would not be the case. Available medical research literature provides support for their conclusions.

Some research shows no long-term effects, and other research results show potential *short-term* forgetfulness in some cases, but not long-lasting. The Alzheimer's Society (based in the United Kingdom) summarized the state of knowledge on these themes. Their website posting stated:

> "Whilst there is a known short-term effect of anaesthesia on memory (called postoperative cognitive decline), studies that have investigated a link between dementia risk and general anesthetics have found mixed results. These inconsistent findings make it difficult to definitively say whether or not general anaesthetics increases risk of dementia."[42]

## Why This Discussion?

If we had been aware of this body of medical research, we could have initiated discussions with our neurological and addiction treatment teams about the timing of Nancy's menopause and her surgical history. Such information may have been helpful in developing diagnosis and treatment plans for Nancy. In any event, my readers may find these topics relevant to their situations.

This summary is no substitute for professional opinions by your healthcare and addiction treatment teams. I only suggest that you discuss your loved one's menopausal timing and surgical histories so that they can apply up-to-date medical research findings appropriate to your loved one's circumstances.

# Part 3

## Adjusting to the New Normal: 2013-2014

# Chapter 12

# The Four Jobs of Being a Caregiver

## Juggling Demands of Four Jobs

As Nancy's diagnosis, medical referrals, and addiction treatments progressed, I held at least four jobs.

My first job was my salaried professional position, which I thankfully could perform at home along with frequent business trips lasting one to four days. I liked my work, and my supervisors were understanding of my situation. I had flexibility to address my household needs while also fulfilling my employer's and clients' expectations.

My second job was being Nancy's *de facto* guardian: tracking and scheduling Nancy's medical appointments, coping with continual uncertainties and the "clean up" of whatever occurred while she was drinking, preparing meals, asking our private social worker to undertake specific tasks to support Nancy, and addressing our legal and financial planning needs. I was not a caregiver in the sense of feeding or bathing a frail elder, but I was "Planner-in-Chief" to keep the household and our lives stable. I was on call 24/7 because I never knew what would occur in the next hour (for example, a car crash, or a stove burner left on).

My third job was maintaining my physical and mental health. I continued my regime of daily workouts at our community fitness center, or I ran three to four miles every day. I looked forward to my daily gym workouts and my runs because they boosted both my physical stamina and my state of mind. I took periodic weekend breaks out-of-town for a change of scenery. Sometimes, I added a day or two to my business trips when I could spend a few days with out-of-state friends. Members of our Alzheimer's Association local chapter support group told me to take care of myself; otherwise, both Nancy and I would decline.

One day I decided to call James, one of my best friends, with whom I had not spoken for two years. I wanted to update him on our situation and ask him about his wife. James was not easy to reach; he did not embrace email, and he had a hearing deficit so he may or may not hear a ringing phone. He retired after selling his partnership stake in a consulting firm, but James spent much of his retirement caring for his wife, Joan. While performing a minor repair of a ceiling fan in their Front Range (Colorado) mountain cabin, Joan suffered an apparent seizure and fell from a seven feet tall ladder on which she was standing. She suffered significant head trauma from which she never recovered. James and Joan were devoted to each other, loved to travel, and had been looking forward to a long retirement together.

In an earlier call, James described Joan's increasing time sleeping and her inability to engage in the world around her. As a caregiver himself, James advised, "You need to take care of yourself, Karl!"

Before I placed my long-deferred call with James, I wanted to be prepared for the likelihood that Joan had passed due to her extensive head injuries. For several hours, I searched the online archives in all the local newspapers in their metropolitan area looking for Joan's obituary.

*Unfortunately, I did not find her obituary, but I found his. James had died.*

James was a tragic example of the caregiver passing before his loved one. The support group's insights were far too accurate. I was heartbroken. The four of us had spent so many wonderful times together. They had been among our best and longest adult friends after college. Now James had died, Joan was unreachable, and I felt a great emptiness.

My fourth job was working with Beth, my sister, to support our 80-year-old mother and monitor her health and living circumstances. Beth and I were and still are quite close, and we worked well together in supporting Mom. Dad died at 86 years old from a heart attack during a holiday weekend. After the funeral, Beth and I stepped in to help Mom maintain the house for two years, address her legal and financial matters, and supply other support. We took turns visiting her and organizing her progressive elder care needs. She lived over 1,800 miles away from Beth and me, so addressing her needs was a challenge. She would not move closer to us. Beth and I each had our own to-do list to address, which we coordinated. Dad's many deferred home maintenance issues were paramount, so we needed to arrange for remodeling and repair contractors. Seasonal service providers were also needed, like lawnmowers and snow shovelers.

When Mom told us she was ready to move into a nearby senior apartment, we helped her move and we readied the house for sale. Five years later we helped her move into a nursing home. Beth was also supportive of me as I sought to find proper treatment and care for Nancy. I could not ask for a better sister.

## From Husband to Caregiver

I had been Nancy's best friend, and she had been mine. We had our lives' pathways charted, and even with normal life challenges, we were committed to staying together. We had supported one another throughout our thirty-plus years. I was determined to help Nancy overcome her hurdles with alcohol abuse and WKS to restore our earlier relationship of love and support. However, since I was on the receiving end of her drunken stupors and deception, I took the advice of my fellow caregivers to maintain my health and my life. If she did not want a life, then I was still going to have one. But along the way, I would help her get the support she needed.

The years-long demands from coping with Nancy's alcohol abuse and the effects of WKS were draining; my days were filled with sadness, urgency, frustration, joylessness, and knowing on a day-to-day basis that I had to do it all. For a while, Nancy could still shop for groceries, run errands, help with laundry, and perform simple cooking tasks. But as her alcoholism progressed (and later, as her Korsakoff's

Syndrome condition progressed), increasingly I bore more household and care responsibilities.

I cannot describe the despair and stress that comes from the lack of control in living with an adult who may do harm to herself or to others. In my world, the uncertainties and demands were relentless, and the stakes were high. There was no one else to help me day-to-day. It was just me and Nancy.

## My Mental Health

In the mid-1970s, after I graduated from my master's program, I suffered from depression when I could not find a job and Nancy's position was eliminated due to budget constraints. After I found a job, I gave no further thought to this initial bout of depression.

However, in the mid-1980s I again suffered depression after I moved to New England to rejoin Nancy after an informal, eighteen-month separation. I entered therapy with Katherine, a family and marriage counselor, and her husband, Dr. Ralph, who was a psychiatrist. In addition to my therapy with Katherine, I had periodic therapy sessions with her husband who prescribed an antidepressant (AD) which I took for about six months. Together with my therapy sessions with Katherine and Dr. Ralph, along with the AD med, I worked through the depression.

Now, twenty years later, amid my challenges with Nancy, I was back in Katherine's therapy room. Thankfully, she was still in practice and welcomed me back. She helped me to find ways of coping and staying sane as I balanced all my responsibilities stemming from Nancy's alcohol abuse and Korsakoff's Syndrome.

Katherine knew that I had a Type-A personality and I always tended to tackle work projects directed my way. I was exhausted physically and mentally from both my job and personal responsibilities at home. Katherine coached me to pause and then consider the actual priority of the many job assignments and requests which were directed at me. For example, she extolled the virtues of procrastination: "Karl, procrastinators can be very successful people."

Katherine also told me to be kind to myself: "You have major burdens, and you are managing these burdens very well." I did not always feel that way, especially on those days when I could only focus *one minute at a time* to get something done. I had so many incoming missiles from my four jobs, the responsibilities were overwhelming, and my head spun. I slowly progressed to being able to work – without panicking – for five-minute periods, then fifteen minutes, then an hour, and eventually back to something approaching normalcy. Parents, especially single parents, undoubtedly understand this well.

In addition to weekly therapy, Katherine referred me to another psychiatrist, Dr. Marc, for therapy and appropriate medications. (Katherine's husband had retired.) Together, Dr. Marc and Katherine helped me cope with my demands and ordeals.

My parents and ancestors were stoic and resourceful people, who lived through the Great Depression, two world wars and several European wars, famine, and more. Even in mid-twentieth-century America, seeking mental health care was not something you did lightly, and you certainly would not share this fact with anyone else. But I needed this help, and so had my mother. She fought depression and anxiety throughout her life.

Reaching out for mental health assistance is important when you need it. I told friends about my therapy. I was not and am not ashamed. Just like physical health, mental health is essential for a full life.

## Serenity Prayer

One afternoon, shortly after Nancy's diagnosis with WKS, I entered Katherine's therapy room eager to ask her three burning existential questions: *"Why is this happening to us? Why this tragedy? How can a loving God allow for such pain and agony?"*

Katherine pulled a book from her office bookshelf and gave it to me. Harold Kushner, in his book *When Bad Things Happen to Good People,*[43] approached my questions from a theological viewpoint. Being raised in a conservative branch of a Protestant church denomination, this book was a good beginning to help me answer my questions.

Kushner's bottom-line message was quite clear: *Bad things happen to good people, and good things happen to bad people. Life is unfair.* I viewed his messages within the context of the Old Testament of the Bible: The human condition stemmed from Original Sin. From the moment in Paradise when Adam and Eve – with free will – chose to eat the fruit of the Tree of Good and Evil, thereby disobeying God, Paradise was lost. Humankind had chosen poorly and was banished to inequity, suffering, and pain.

I was satisfied and comforted by Kushner's book. *You are not alone. Suffering and inequity are found everywhere.* His book also reminded me to live by the Serenity Prayer[44] by accepting what I can change, recognizing what I cannot change, and understanding the difference.

Therapy, in its many forms, has been an important part of responding to the demands of caregiving in the context of alcohol abuse and Korsakoff's Syndrome. Later in this book, we will explore additional therapy approaches for trauma and moving on from trauma.

# Chapter 13

# Progression

## Sundowning

Not long after receiving Nancy's first diagnosis of Korsakoff's, I observed an alarming new behavior. While she was mostly alert, coherent, and active from morning to mid-afternoon, around 4:00 PM she became forgetful and unfocused. I could not have a conversation with her. By now, I was well-read about dementia and aware of the late-afternoon phenomena known as sundowning, when dementia patients lose focus and have diminished capabilities. Seeing these behaviors in Nancy, I concluded she was experiencing sundowning.

Two weeks later at our monthly dementia support group meeting, I described my observations of Nancy's likely sundowning behaviors to my fellow caregivers and volunteer facilitators. They concurred that the behavior she exhibited did indeed mirror their experiences with sundowning. I took my observations of these behaviors as a sign that her condition was deteriorating, and I planned to inform her neurological team by phone or at our upcoming follow-up neurological evaluation.

However, I soon learned Nancy's sundowning was not what it seemed. She was not abstaining; she was still drinking. While I was working upstairs in my home office, Nancy was drinking out of my sight downstairs in our family room. This behavior worsened after she lost her consulting contracts and she had little to do.

I discovered her surreptitious drinking for several days in a row around 3:30-4:00 PM. I walked from my upstairs office through the kitchen to our family room. I discovered emptied or half-emptied bottles of vodka, other spirits, or wine on the kitchen counter that she inadvertently left out. In the family room, I saw ice-cube-filled glass tumblers holding Nancy's vodka which she set beside her on the chair's side table, or sometimes on the floor as she tried to keep the glasses out of my sight.

Nancy was adamant that she was not drinking, and she played the role of teetotaler while consuming both non-alcoholic beer and wine in front of me. Bottom-line: Nancy was certainly not sundowning.

---

**TWO TELLTALE SIGNS OF KORSAKOFF'S**

Patients with Korsakoff's have no self-awareness that they are affected. This lack of self-awareness and confabulation create challenges for spouses, families, and caregivers because patients will object to addiction treatment and other actions to treat or accommodate their memory loss.

Based on my experience and study results in medical peer-reviewed literature, as soon as you observe these conditions plus apathy and gait changes, you may wish to consult with your medical care teams. If WKS is diagnosed early, treatment and abstinence may lead to some memory reversal.

---

## She Seems OK to Me: Confabulation

Nancy had been telling mutual friends that I was making much ado about nothing regarding her alcohol abuse and memory loss. During errands at local grocery stores or restaurants, or occasionally at a neighborhood gathering, people would sometimes take me aside and say, "Gee, Nancy seems OK to me. It looks like she is doing fine."

But after fifteen minutes or so, they too observed Nancy repeating the same stories in the same conversation as if she had never uttered those words, or she would spin a story that had no basis in truth.

This was confabulation, where dementia patients involuntarily fill-in memory gaps. Both confabulation and the patient's lack of self-awareness of their situation are well documented in medical literature as being signs of Korsakoff's.

## Relationship of Memory to Everyday Life

The creation of, and access to, memories depend on neurological processes in specific areas of the brain.[45] We all draw upon these processes to recall those great moments watching the sunset across the Grand Canyon from the South Rim, your daughter's garden wedding, or perhaps Uncle Fred's stale joke that he repeated at each Thanksgiving dinner. When specific areas of the brain are damaged by alcohol and/or thiamine deficiency (such as they are through Wernicke's Encephalopathy and Korsakoff's Syndrome), the brain's ability to create and recall memories is disrupted.

We draw upon our memory for *every task* we undertake. When I say, "I'll take my shower before breakfast," you and I perceive this task as one action – taking a shower. But in fact, it is a series of small discrete tasks – disrobing, opening the shower door or curtain, turning on the water flow using the faucet handle, walking into the shower, closing the door, lathering the shampoo, rinsing, using hair conditioner, grabbing a bar of soap, washing the body, rinsing, turning off the water, exiting the shower, closing the curtain or closing the shower door, and finally drying ourselves.

You and I take for granted our routine ability to perform these actions. In fact, we just think of it as one task. We learned how to perform each step of taking a shower or bath early in our lives and it is stored in our memory. When we want to take a shower, we just do it seamlessly and we unconsciously tap our memory for *each* step.

However, for a loved one with reduced cognitive function, taking a shower or washing the dishes or any other aspect of living may become increasingly difficult. People with dementia simply cannot access the memory to recall each step, so eventually, a caregiver needs to prompt them and, even later, perform the task with them. A caregiver must assist the person to prepare for the shower. As their dementia progresses, the caregiver may need to bathe them, too. For those with dementia, the ability to perform tasks independently without cues diminishes over time and eventually affects everything a person with dementia tries to do.

When Nancy forgot the three ingredients in the beef stew (noted earlier), it was clear that she was losing the capability to perform some tasks. She would also forget she had just consumed alcohol. For example, after drinking several glasses of wine, she might say, "I think I'll have my first glass of wine before dinner."

Nancy had always prided herself on being quite independent and capable of household and car maintenance. For example, Nancy led our home's landscaping chores and made runs to the local nursery to keep our home's heavily vegetated one-third-acre lot immaculate. Her capability to perform these and other tasks diminished over time.

## The Carport

One moonless night, I returned home just before midnight from a Chicago business trip. I paid the taxi driver, hopped out of the airport taxicab, walked up the dark driveway, entered the silent house through the kitchen sliding glass door, placed my luggage and brief case in the guest room, and went directly to bed in our master bedroom. Early the next morning, I donned my gym gear in our spare bedroom, grabbed a cup of coffee, closed the kitchen door, and walked to our green Subaru to drive to the gym – my usual routine.

As I walked around the car parked in the driveway, I shook my head in disbelief when I saw the damaged driver-side panels, door, and side-view mirror. I then spun around and saw a severed carport support column, leaving one support column. In shock, I reentered the house, and I awoke Nancy to ask what happened. "Oh, yeah, I had a little trouble parking yesterday afternoon," she mumbled and fell back asleep.

While I was relieved that she was not injured nor was anyone else, this was yet another troubling incident that illustrated that her alcoholism and WKS were affecting her ability to function independently and safely. This carport incident resulted in a $4,000 bill from our contractor who rushed to our house that morning to install a temporary support column before the carport collapsed. The next day, he installed a new permanent support beam, repaired collateral damage, and painted the new timbers. Fortunately for us, he was available, and we averted a collapsed carport. But our car insurance premium also increased again.

A year later, I sold our Subaru to a nationally recognized used-car dealer. During the transaction, the dealership's buying agent pointed to the spot where damage from the carport incident had been repaired. I could not really argue with him. Upon closer inspection, I could also see that the repair was quite visible, and the quality of the repair was substandard. He then handed me a check for $3,000 less than the average Kelly Blue Book value.

Nancy's run-in with the carport support column cost over $7,000 in total, plus the car repair costs. This was but one example of the energy-draining series of never-ending household disruptions, new expenses, and constant surprises.

## The Futility of Checking-In

During my extensive business travel, I usually called Nancy in the late afternoon or evening from my hotel room to say hello, ask her about her day, discuss socializing plans, and coordinate household chores. I might ask, "What's the latest on the contractor's bid to replace the windows?" or "Did the landscapers replace the bush in the corner of the house near the family room window?" or "Could you please call Gary and Suzette to confirm our arrival time for dinner on Saturday?" Every day around the world, tens of millions of such exchanges undoubtedly occur between spouses, partners, and family members.

As Nancy's drinking increased and her cognitive impairment progressed due to Korsakoff's Syndrome, these telephone exchanges morphed into futile exercises. Upon my return home, I would ask about the status of the tasks we had discussed on the phone. Sometimes my questions would be met with blank stares, or worse. She might tell me, "No, I didn't call the contractor. Sorry." But when I called, the contractor said, "Oh, Nancy already called and we're taking care of it." Or the reverse would happen – she would tell me she called Frank, but in fact, she had not. Increasingly, I never knew the truth from untruths or action from inaction. *Everything had to be verified.*

Over time, I was lucky if she even answered the phone when I called. When she would answer, her slurred words betrayed her drinking. Early one Sunday afternoon, upon arrival at a conference hotel in St. Louis, I needed to speak with Nancy about a household matter. I called her as I waited to be served my late lunch order. Unfortunately, when she answered the phone, her incoherence at once betrayed her early drinking. Nancy was already inebriated and incapable of holding a phone conversation with me.

These calls home during my business trips were pointless, and they only made me anxious and frustrated. I stopped calling.

Between the alcohol and the cognitive impairment from Korsakoff's, Nancy and I could no longer have meaningful communication. In a close relationship, couples take such phone calls for granted. They keep us connected. In real-time, we hear about the joys and tribulations of work or home life or share funny travel stories with our spouse or partner. In my situation, that all ended. The connective tissue between two friends was fraying, and our bonds unraveling.

Besides the sadness and frustration caused by these pointless calls, the consequence of Nancy's inability to act on household matters in my absence meant that more tasks fell on me. The mental and physical burdens increased. I lost weight and reverted to my appearance as a scrawny high school teenager. Nancy and I were isolated from our friends and from one another. I was losing (or had already lost) Nancy.

# Chapter 14

# Uncertainty and Confabulation

## Uncertainty

In the previous chapter, I noted the challenges of calling Nancy during business trips. But the challenges of her confabulation and uncertainty extended far beyond phone calls. Uncertainty is one of the most energy-draining and spirit-sapping aspects of living with a highly functioning adult alcoholic with Korsakoff's Syndrome.

I could not truly relax at home. I never knew, for example, when Nancy would start drinking early in the day. Would we have a "normal" day? Would the day and evening disintegrate with her early drinking? Would she return from an errand with yet more car damage, or even worse, had she hit something or someone? Would she pass or fail the urine test at her addiction treatment center? Would she pass out after dinner before we could resolve an issue or address a household need?

My days devolved into a game of chess, where I needed to constantly monitor and anticipate her moves. But unlike my past casual enjoyment of chess, this was not a game.

## Lying or Confabulation?

Earlier, I mentioned the challenge of needing to verify Nancy's actions and statements when I introduced confabulation. Living with someone with Korsakoff's is not only challenging, but it is also frightening. As the Alzheimer's Association web page explains:

> "Those with Korsakoff syndrome may 'confabulate,' or make up, information they can't remember. They are not 'lying' but may believe their invented explanations. Scientists don't yet understand the mechanism by which Korsakoff syndrome may cause confabulation. The person may also see or hear things that are not there (hallucinations)."[46]

I had to question and verify Nancy's statements of fact. Verification was necessary to maintain her health and safety, as well as my own, and to protect our property as well as our community. Verification became a vital part of my routine job as a caregiver.

With no real treatment options and Nancy's continued drinking, tension increasingly filled our home. We were no longer blessed with the nurturing, intimate, mutually supportive relationship that we once had. Our relationship deteriorated with every passing week. My hope for the successful reversal of her condition diminished too.

## Unreliable

In late 2013, my ophthalmologist and eye surgeon agreed I needed cataract surgery in one eye. This surgery was scheduled at an outpatient surgery center about a 90-minute (non-rush-hour) drive from our home. We booked a hotel room near the outpatient surgery center for two nights. The procedure was scheduled for 7:00 AM on the first day, and there was a 24-hour post-op exam on the second day at 10:00 AM at the eye surgeon's office.

The procedure was successfully performed in fifteen minutes, with about an hour of paperwork and pre-op and an hour of post-op time. The outpatient surgery center released me before lunch. Back at the hotel, I needed to rest from our early rising. I was hungry because I had to fast for twelve hours before the procedure. I fell into bed to rest and recover, but before dozing off around 11:30 AM, I asked Nancy to obtain lunch for us at a deli, which was a five-minute walk from our hotel. After reviewing the online menu with my good eye, I placed my lunch order with her, and off she went. I awoke an hour later, and

Nancy had not yet returned. Still no Nancy after 75 minutes.

Finally, between 1:15-1:30 PM, she appeared with the food. "Well, they seemed to have mixed up the order. They had to remake everything. That's why this took so long for me to return," she explained.

Despite my groggy recovery from sedation, I was suspicious about Nancy's delayed return. No doubt, she had consumed one or two quick drinks at the deli or a nearby restaurant – the real reason for her delay. My suspicions were later confirmed that night at dinner when Nancy complained of feeling nauseous. "I'm sick to my stomach," she said as she picked at her now-unappetizing plate of food. After our late lunch, she made a show in our hotel room of taking a dose of her Antabuse® prescription designed to cause nausea from alcohol. Because we were not drinking any alcoholic beverages at dinner, her nausea at dinner confirmed that she had been drinking while making the lunch run.

I was at my wit's end. I thought to myself, *"She can't even stay sober when I need her to be a caregiver. I can't trust her to manage any important matters."*

Nancy needed to stop drinking, but traditional addiction treatment was ineffective due to the complication of Korsakoff's Syndrome. With my job, I could not watch her 24/7 to impose abstinence. Absent any further ideas from our support and medical teams, I thought intervention by a psychiatrist with a specialty in treating patients with Korsakoff's Syndrome might help Nancy "get it" and guide her to abstinence. But that search had to wait for Nancy's upcoming second comprehensive neurological assessment.

# Chapter 15

# Second Neurological Evaluation

## One Year Return

A year after Nancy's first neuropsychological testing and diagnosis, we were once again seated in the neurology center's waiting room on a grayish, damp early summer day. Since the first assessment, Nancy entered residential alcohol addiction treatment and was released after one month. After entering two intensive outpatient treatment centers, she was terminated from both. She was non-compliant; she consistently failed their drug tests for alcohol. While we had acted on the key recommendation from the first evaluation test results, she did not or could not abstain.

Nancy's second round of neuropsychological assessment tests followed the same sequence as the previous year, although with a different neuropsychologist, Dr. Rogers. We spent the evening before the tests at a nearby hotel to ensure Nancy was rested upon arrival at the clinic and not delayed by morning rush-hour traffic. The testing day started with a short consultation at 9:00 AM with Dr. Rogers, followed by Nancy's morning tests, lunch break, afternoon tests, and release at 4:00 PM in time to battle rush-hour traffic with a hazy sun in my eyes.

When staff led Nancy into the testing room, I spent one-to-one time with Dr. Rogers. I shared my observations that Nancy's cognition had declined. Also, I noted her continued drinking even though she was going through the motions of consuming only non-alcoholic wine and beer. I told Dr. Rogers that Nancy had entered a residential and two outpatient addiction treatment centers, was released from the residential facility after one month, and was later terminated by the two outpatient centers for non-compliance (failing the blood tests for alcohol). I told her of three addiction treatment therapists' pessimism about Nancy fully embracing her situation but that I was still hopeful that we could somehow support Nancy to help her find a pathway to abstinence. Dr. Rogers listened attentively and asked clarifying questions before she moved on to supervise and conduct a repeat of Nancy's day-long testing protocol.

We waited four weeks to receive a call from Dr. Rogers' office to schedule our review of her test results. In the now-familiar neuropsychological unit's consultation room, Dr. Rogers reviewed the results where she affirmed that Nancy registered a slight decline in cognition – barely statistically significant, but nonetheless, Nancy had not improved.

Nancy sat quietly with a set jaw and tight lips and then rationalized her performance when she told Dr. Rogers, "I didn't really get a good night's sleep before the tests."

Nancy's original diagnosis was confirmed, and Dr. Rogers' assessment mirrored the earlier evaluation, especially Nancy's lack of awareness of her memory problems. Dr. Rogers reported that Nancy was high functioning in social and verbal skills (very characteristic of Korsakoff's Syndrome patients) but exhibited confabulation where she would automatically and unconsciously fill in her memory gaps. Dr. Rogers observed that Nancy's social and verbal skills could give a casual observer the impression that she did not have cognitive impairment. She also noted that Nancy denied her memory challenges and continued to believe my concerns were overblown. Dr. Rogers said Nancy was clinically deficient in self-awareness.

In closing, Dr. Rogers gave us five sobering recommendations. First, Nancy needed external 24/7 oversight to restrict her alcohol consumption. This should be done through stays in an extended, specialized inpatient residential treatment or another type of facility. Without such oversight, Dr. Rogers believed Nancy was unlikely to control her alcohol consumption by herself.

Second, Dr. Rogers said further neuropsychological evaluations should not be performed unless there were significant new circumstances.

Dr. Rogers then closed out our session with three more recommendations: schedule a formal driving assessment, install breathalyzer interlock systems in both cars, and adjust Nancy's day-to-day life to provide greater regularity to her schedule (for example, daily planning, avoiding multitasking, and organizing household items).

I was puzzled. Dr. Rogers had confirmed Nancy's lack of sufficient self-awareness to cease drinking on her own and that she lacked insights to acknowledge she had memory impairment. Yet Dr. Rogers said Nancy should re-enter residential addiction treatment to abstain to prevent further cognitive decline. But how could this be achieved?

Our options seemed quite limited. Nancy couldn't stop drinking herself, and she lacked self-awareness. So, how would Nancy be helped by placing her in the specialized residential addiction treatment center? With her lack of self-awareness, how would that help when she left? That money would be wasted. To make matters worse, I could not provide 24/7 oversight since I was still working and traveling, nor could we afford in-home personnel to perform that oversight in my absence.

I could not envision a sustainable path forward, and unfortunately, Dr. Rogers offered no alternative suggestions other than a heartfelt wish that Nancy's endeavor to abstain would be successful. The lingering question was whether she could or would stop herself with the lack of self-awareness noted by our neurological team and the staff of the three addiction treatment programs in which Nancy had participated.

## Neurologist Follow-up Appointment

Soon, we were back in Nancy's neurologist's office, where Dr. Edwards reviewed the test results of Nancy's second neurological assessment.

She emphasized that Nancy was depleting her cognitive reserve. Nancy was now in danger of progressing to a more serious loss of cognition, including the possibility of Alzheimer's Disease in addition to advancing Korsakoff's Syndrome.

Dr. Edwards added that there was no immediate need for any other follow-up appointments with her or their neuropsychologists unless Nancy showed a noticeable change in behavior or if other alarming symptoms appeared. She repeated his warnings about the impact of alcohol on her brain function. Nancy sat emotionless. Dr. Edwards offered no additional options about how we might move forward.

Our somber drive home was mostly in silence. I was lost in thought about how or whether to try to place Nancy in yet another addiction treatment or how we could cost-effectively isolate her from access to alcohol. However, we now needed to act on each of the five recommendations of Drs. Jones and Edwards.

# Chapter 16

# Perils and Management of Driving

## Driving Tests

Given the potential property and personal injury risks from Nancy's continued driving, I first acted upon the neurological team's recommendation to evaluate Nancy's driving skills. With reluctance and defiance, Nancy agreed to take a driver-evaluation test. She viewed it as a challenge to me and her doctors – "I know I'm a good driver, but I'll do this to satisfy all of you," she said as we walked into the test center.

The evaluation consisted of written, oral, and on-the-road tests. Her evaluation consumed the entire day. In the late afternoon, Nancy and the testing lead staff member appeared from the testing rooms, and the staff member said, "Nancy passed all the tests." I was incredulous, and Nancy gloated at the news, "See, Karl, I told you I could pass this!" The staff told us they were surprised, too, but she passed all the tests, including on-the-road tests. I thought to myself as we walked back to our car, "*Well, those results didn't turn out the way I expected.*"

I had mixed feelings about Nancy's driving-test results. Yes, she could still legally drive for local errands after I installed the breathalyzer interlock systems. Because I was often on business travel, her ability to drive would certainly be convenient. However, as Nancy grew more forgetful, often drove erratically, and had damaged our carport and her car, I was terrified of her diminished ability to avoid collisions with other cars, objects, and pedestrians. Second, I was also concerned about her safety. Third, I was concerned about our potential personal legal and financial liabilities if she caused personal injuries and property damage.

Taken as a whole, her driving abilities were disturbing. I needed to address the neurological center's recommendation to remove our remaining vehicles from our house or install breathalyzers in our two cars.[47]

---

**MANAGING DRIVING RISKS**

Addressing your loved one's ability to drive will not likely be an easy matter for you and your loved one to resolve. However, the personal liability and public safety concerns are too great to ignore the questions of whether your loved one should continue driving or not. In our case, our neurological clinic had driving skills evaluation capabilities in-house. You may wish to ask your neurology team for a referral if they do not have in-house capabilities.

---

## Installing Ignition Breathalyzers

I collected information about breathalyzer ignition interlock equipment, installation requirements and costs, recurring monthly charges, and required maintenance activities and costs (including monthly calibration of the breathalyzer).

I decided to donate our oldest vehicle, an older-model Nissan Maxima, to the Kars 4 Kids volunteer organization. With only one car, we limited Nancy's vehicular access and reduced our costs for installing and maintaining breathalyzer ignition interlock systems.

I was now ready to sign my contract with a breathalyzer ignition interlock system vendor and schedule training and the installation in our Subaru, our only remaining car. But a day before my planned call to sign the contract, we received a bombshell letter that rendered these actions unnecessary.

## A Godsend

In March 2014, Nancy received a letter from our state's Department of Motor Vehicles (DMV). Unbeknownst to us, the driving test center was required by state law to send Nancy's test results to the state DMV along with a full report containing the reasons for Nancy's driving test. The test center reported Nancy's diagnosis of Korsakoff's Syndrome and her cognitive impairment, which in turn triggered DMV's license-revocation letter to Nancy. The letter stated: As of April 1, 2014, Nancy was prohibited from driving due to her cognitive impairment.

This directive was great news. First, the prohibition would keep her safe as well as the driving and pedestrian public and others' property. Second, her removal from driving would help to protect our assets from lawsuits. Nancy and I discussed the seriousness of this requirement, and I reinforced that she could no longer drive. She would need to either walk, ask neighbors for help, or arrange transportation with Susan, our private social worker.

## Complication

With this DMV order, I assumed Nancy would stop driving the Subaru and that she would be driven to medical appointments and errands either by our private social worker or friends or she would use taxis and car-sharing services when I was out of town. Therefore, I did not install the breathalyzer as I thought Nancy would follow the state order and she would leave our remaining car in the driveway for my use.

I told Susan about the DMV order and asked two sets of neighbors to keep an eye on Nancy's compliance. Several weeks later, neighbors told me that Nancy was still driving when I was gone. I called my attorney the next day to tell him about the DMV letter and our neighbors' reports of Nancy's continued driving. He was blunt.

He said I could be named in a civil lawsuit if Nancy crashed the car, and that crash resulted in personal injuries and/or property damage. "The plaintiffs' attorney would tell the court that your name was still on the car's title and registration. Second, you knew she was an alcoholic and was cognitively impaired with Korsakoff's Syndrome. Third, you knew she was still driving. Lastly, you did not take any reasonable steps to prevent her from driving while intoxicated."

My attorney's guidance left me with no choice. I rented a space at a nearby self-storage-unit complex to park our remaining car. Now, only I had access to the Subaru. This action solved two issues: Nancy could no longer drive, and I did not have to install the ignition interlock system.

# Chapter 17

## Our New Medical Professional

After we received the results of Nancy's second neurological assessment and I had addressed two priority needs (the driving assessment, and the breathalyzer installation), I could again focus on locating a psychiatrist with experience in treating patients with Korsakoff's Syndrome.

I soon found a psychiatrist with the desired experience. I contacted Dr. Roberts by phone and explained Nancy's alcohol abuse and her WKS diagnosis, and he agreed to an initial consultation.

During the initial session, Dr. Roberts first gave me a few minutes of private time. I reviewed the situation from my perspective, supplied a brief history of Nancy's alcohol abuse, and related Nancy's diagnosis and addiction treatment. I also shared my hopes and aspirations for a turn-around and my despair and disappointment with the trends in Nancy's behavior and condition. I also related the dire warnings from Drs. Jones and Edwards about Nancy's further cognitive decline and Nancy's continued drinking.

Dr. Roberts then saw Nancy alone. At the conclusion of this first consultation, Dr. Roberts agreed to accept Nancy as a patient.

Nancy had several subsequent appointments with Dr. Roberts. Since I was still engaged in significant business travel, Susan (our private social worker) sometimes ferried Nancy to these and other appointments. During this time, Dr. Roberts also consulted with another neurologist and a psychiatrist from another renowned medical center.

The results of these consultations with Dr. Roberts and the other specialists were disappointing. Nancy exhibited no discernable change in her drinking behavior. I had hoped Dr. Roberts might help Nancy in some way to breakthrough her denials, but these consultations were either ineffective or simply too late. Nancy's cognitive impairment had now presumably progressed to the point that she was unable to change on her own, as her neurological team had concluded in their second assessment results.

Except for thiamine therapy, which was of limited value because Nancy continued to drink, it seemed clear to me now that no injections, surgery, medicines, or therapy could restore Nancy's lost cognition or convert her to practicing abstinence. Nancy needed to abstain from alcohol, which was unlikely, or I needed to place her in a setting of forced abstinence such as an assisted living or other care facility.

## Additional Residential Treatment?

We had been along this pathway of neurological diagnosis and addiction treatment for two and a half years. Nancy had been terminated by the two intensive outpatient addiction treatment centers, she still drank, and the neurological team recommended either extended residential treatment or other ways to isolate Nancy from alcohol so she might recover modest cognitive function. She was not attending AA and was continuing her heavy drinking, either by choice or due to an inability to control herself.

None of our professional medical team, the addiction treatment centers, the Alzheimer Association, or anyone else had ideas for what I should do besides placing Nancy in the ultra-expensive specialized residential treatment at a Florida facility. Placing Nancy in a high-end treatment facility for months seemed fruitless. Without self-awareness, she would resume her drinking upon exiting the facility.

## What's Next?

I was at a loss. I tried to think of another pathway, both for Nancy to somehow achieve a breakthrough with her drinking and how I could still be supportive. I also thought of important guidance from both my Dementia Support Group and the book, *The 36-Hour Day*: Caregivers need to take care of themselves. Caregivers often die before their loved ones.[48]

During a long drive home on a late Sunday afternoon in December 2013, I reflected on the next steps to help Nancy as well as my own future. The weather was melancholy. I drove along a winding state highway through rolling foothills, with skies of sullen winter clouds mixed with struggling rays of fading sunlight that cast dull shadows across the brown fields awaiting spring planting.

Against the backdrop of this moody landscape, I made two decisions. First, I needed to explore *the possibility* of moving out of our home, temporarily or more permanently, either in the area or out of state. I couldn't go on. I was spent physically and mentally from trying to keep my job and cope with Nancy's further decline and worsening alcohol abuse. Second, I realized we still needed to place Nancy in a facility where we might be able to restrict her alcohol access and where she would be amenable to moving to this facility.

# Chapter 18

# Care Option Revisited

## A "New" Option

Following that late December drive, I called Susan (our private social worker) to schedule time with me to revisit Nancy's short-term care needs. Our neurological medical team had been unanimous that Nancy needed a stable living environment where she could be monitored 24/7 and where she would be living in monitored abstinence.

In our discussion, I asked Susan to contact a nearby continuing care retirement community (CCRC). Nancy and I had been on the wait-list for this CCRC, and I said we should apply for Nancy's solo residency. If accepted, I was quite sure Nancy would be willing to move there because of our past application there.

In 2008, Nancy and I applied for residency at this CCRC and had been on their wait list. We sought a two-bedroom end-unit with ample amounts of natural light. It was located at tree level and did not feel like being in an apartment building. These units felt more like small ranch-style houses than an apartment. As expected, these units were in high demand, and turnover was low.

We had carefully planned for financing our move to this CCRC. The sale of our house would have covered the initial entrance fees for both of us.[49] Our combined Social Security payments would cover the monthly fees, and our IRAs/401ks would pay for our day-to-day expenses. It would have been a perfect living solution for us.

As with all CCRCs,[50] residents enter the facility in an independent living apartment which includes one or two meals a day, once-a-week apartment cleaning, and access to other amenities like a fitness center, recreational programs, and more. If a resident later needs assisted living, they are simply moved within the CCRC's property to one of those units. Residents later needing memory care or skilled nursing care would then move into those units (either on-site or at a nearby contracted facility).

CCRCs require that residents stay in independent living for a defined minimum period. While the minimum stay will vary with individual CCRCs according to their individual financial operating requirements, the principal model is the same.[51] The costs to maintain residents in independent living are less than the monthly fee. In other words, the monthly fee is initially under-utilized during a resident's time in independent living. When residents need assisted living or skilled nursing, the monthly costs exceed the monthly payments (over-utilizing services). In the end, the cost and monthly fee revenues are balanced. Residents have the comfort of knowing they pay a flat monthly fee (except for inflationary adjustments), and they can appropriately plan their personal budgets and finances.

Ironically, Nancy and I never moved into this CCRC. We had not cleared their wait list before Nancy's Korsakoff's diagnosis. If we had moved into the CCRC earlier, our situation now would be simple. We would have lived enough time in our independent living unit so that Nancy could be transferred to an assisted living or a memory care unit. I could have remained in our independent living unit.

Now we could not enter the CCRC as a couple and live in separate living levels (me in independent living, and Nancy in assisted living or memory care). We would not satisfy the conditions of their financial model, and I soon learned this constraint applied to Nancy seeking solo residency.

## Seeking CCRC Solo Residency for Nancy

While I was uncertain that the CCRC would accept Nancy alone, I believed it was still worth a try, so I asked Susan to apply to the CCRC for Nancy's solo admittance. The finances would still work well on our side – her half of the future house-sale revenue would pay for her single entrance fee. Her monthly fees would have been paid from benefits from her long-term-care insurance policy, her Social Security benefits, and her IRAs.

Susan contacted the CCRC's intake staff, and we prepared and submitted Nancy's application. In addition to our paperwork, the CCRC administered an assessment of Nancy's living capabilities. These are often called Activities of Daily Life, or ADLs.

We soon learned the results of the CCRCs assessment of Nancy's ADL capabilities and their review of our application. Unfortunately, Nancy was not accepted. She failed to meet their approval review criteria. With Nancy's WKS diagnosis and demonstrated limitations from the neurological assessments, the staff knew Nancy could not remain long, if at all, in an independent living unit. Her steady progression of cognitive impairment would necessitate a near-term transfer into their assisted living or memory care units. Such a quick move would not fit their financial model.

Susan and I were disappointed. The staff at this CCRC were caring people, and the infrastructure and services were outstanding. But we had to accept the fact that they would not accept Nancy. We understood their reasoning, but we were still crushed. This would have been the ideal solution for Nancy's care. This decision, however, left us with no other immediate care possibility for Nancy.

# Part 4

## Transitioning: 2014-2016

# Chapter 19

# The Tipping Point

In early 2014, Nancy had no addiction treatment support, she could not work, and we were still living together in our New England house. Her drinking worsened. The situation was no longer sustainable.

## Welcome Home

On a Wednesday evening in mid-April 2014, I called Nancy from my Chicago hotel room to suggest that she meet me the next day upon my return to New England. We would meet at our nearby commuter rail station, and we would have an early dinner. I thought this might be a good break for both of us. She liked the idea, and we agreed I would first call her when my flight arrived. I would call her again while on the commuter train and meet her at our nearby station. After our rendezvous, we would drive to our favorite Turkish restaurant where we often ate lunch or dinner. After settling into our usual booth, our favorite server would ask, "The same tonight, Mr. Karl? Two kofta kebab platters with two soups on the side?"

Nancy did not answer her business phone, our home's landline phone, or her business landline when I called her from the airport upon my arrival. "*Well, maybe she's out on her walk, or maybe she's on her way to the station and was running some errands along the way,*" I hoped.

Once on the commuter train, I tried calling her again. My calls to all three phones again went unanswered. As I stepped off the train at our station, Nancy was nowhere to be seen. She was not on the platform, not in front of the station, and not in the "Kiss and Ride" parking area. Nope. No Nancy. I called the three phones again. No responses.

The taxi cabs based at this suburban station were often old and battered and were driven by ill-tempered, battle-worn men and women. I disliked using these cabs, but on this otherwise pleasant April afternoon with no Nancy in sight and her unreachable, these taxis were my only choice. I was tired, nauseated, and frustrated. I muttered to myself, *"Here we go again. What will I find when I open the door to the house? Why do I even bother to try this?"*

After a seemingly endless, uncomfortable ride in the cab, I arrived at our house. Upon entry, I was met with silence. An empty vodka bottle on the kitchen countertop greeted me. Moving further into the house, I saw Nancy slumped over in my easy chair in the corner of the family room by the window. Backlighting from the late afternoon sun illuminated her crystal cocktail glass sitting on the end table, half-filled with melting ice and vodka.

I asked, "Where have you been? Why didn't you answer the phone and come to the commuter train station?" She slowly opened her unfocused, glassy eyes, barely able to raise her chin to see me, and silently slumped down again.

Another disappointing welcome home. Once upstairs, I flung my briefcase onto my home office desk chair and similarly tossed my luggage in the guest room. I pulled out a few essential items from my dresser and laid them in the guest bedroom for my upcoming night. I could not stand the thought of sleeping in the same bed. It was over. The years of trying to help her stop drinking, her inability to communicate, and not knowing if/when she might crash the car and injure an innocent child – all of this came to a head on an otherwise normal Thursday afternoon in our quiet suburban New England house. The many fender benders and the carport incident. The $50,000 credit card debt that she hid from me until I discovered it when I needed full financial disclosure for a home remodeling loan. All of it. I was done. This was my breaking point. I needed to escape.

That night, I could only see one workable pathway – *Leave now! Leave this weekend! Go far away!*

Since that Sunday afternoon drive in December, I had toyed with assorted options to move out. Besides the option of leaving town, I could have simply moved into an apartment near a suburban subway station. I could commute to our company's downtown office. Or I could have moved to other cities near one of our company's offices. But I decided to flee to Florida, a state that I had often visited and where Nancy and I once considered for our retirement home.

I do not regret the decision that night to leave our New England house to fly to Florida – given my physical and mental state. It was not a *wrong decision*, but I should have initially stayed nearby in New England. Moving locally would have saved significant travel time and money and, no doubt, would have helped me process my grief and recover physically before entering my next phase. However, I was mentally and physically exhausted from the ten-plus years' ordeal.

Another choice on that mid-April evening would have been to place Nancy into assisted living where she would live in monitored abstinence. That option would have taken weeks, if not months. The courts would have needed significant paperwork with justification because I would be seeking to place her against her will.[52]

My attorneys and I could have presented a persuasive case to the Family Court to issue a decree authorizing her placement in assisted living against her will. The medical and addiction treatment teams' documentation would have underscored Nancy's inability of understanding her situation, that she was in denial of her memory issues, was still drinking, was diagnosed with Korsakoff's, and needed 24/7 oversight.

But the choice to place Nancy in assisted living would not have resulted in any immediate change or relief. I could have called my attorney and explored the planning and legal processes for expedited placement in assisted living. However, I did not consult with legal counsel.

Yet another possibility would have been for me to have stayed in a nearby hotel room for a week or more to pause and more thoughtfully consider some longer-term options. But *all I could see that night was escape.*

After all the years of stress, uncertainty, and demands, I was unable to envision other options that night. Moreover, I also naively thought the shock of my moving to a distant location might have jolted Nancy into seeking help. (Spoiler alert: Leaving the house did not have that intended result.)

## Final Arrangements

On Friday morning (after a sleepless night), I told Nancy I was moving out on Sunday. The next two days were a blur. In addition to packing and shipping important papers and clothes, I informed my boss of my plans and obtained his consent, told neighbors, and called and emailed close friends. When my airport shuttle arrived to whisk me to the airport, I doubt Nancy grasped the reality of the situation. She said, "See you when you get back," obviously believing this was a typical business trip.

Upon arrival at the airport, I hustled through TSA Pre-Check security and continued to my concourse. Soon we were in the air. I refined my to-do list for my first few weeks in Florida. I relaxed enough to get a bit of sleep. Upon landing, I felt a knot in my stomach. I was stepping into a new life, and I felt uncertain about how all of this would unfold. I also knew it would take at least a year to legally separate from Nancy and another year to finalize the divorce. Moreover, I suspected Nancy would need a permanent living situation. I doubted she could live alone in our house much longer. Undoubtedly, I would be back in New England again soon.

## Kickoff

Upon arrival, I stayed in a hotel near Tampa International Airport for three nights. This had been a big step. While I was exhausted from the previous 72 hours, I only slept fitfully that first night. Three days later, I moved to an extended-stay hotel within a short drive of the airport to facilitate my business travel. This move would give me time to sort-out longer term housing.

I took personal leave from my job for my first week in Florida so I could locate initial services (like dry cleaners), retrieve my initial UPS shipment of essential business and personal records, and obtain personal and remote office supplies. I then resumed my full-time job, now working remotely from the extended stay and in previously scheduled business travel.

Interspersed with this new beginning, I worked with my first New England attorney to initiate the formal separation agreement and begin addressing other near-term and long-term legal matters. Working with Susan (our private social worker), we aligned on her activities to support Nancy's living arrangements and care. These challenges are described in the next four chapters.

# Chapter 20

# The Dreaded Call

With the CCRC option unavailable, Nancy continued to live in our New England house while I lived in Florida. During my occasional visits in the spring and early summer to retrieve my belongings, I found only limited quantities of food in her refrigerator and pantry. Without a car, Nancy either walked to the nearby grocery store or was driven by a neighbor or our social worker, Susan. Unfortunately, a liquor store was located next to the grocery store, and that was Nancy's continued source of spirits and wine.

I knew Nancy's solo living in our house was temporary, but I needed to develop a solution to keep her safe and healthy. Nancy's care link was Susan, our social worker. We spoke often, and we talked about options after the CCRC had rejected Nancy's application. A solution was not immediately clear, but in the meantime, I asked Susan to continue to support Nancy in our house on her own for as long as possible and to vet potential living options for Nancy.

## The Dreaded Call

The dreaded call came on a Tuesday night in mid-August 2014, around 10:00 PM Eastern time, just shy of four months after I moved out. Our long-time, ever-helpful next-door neighbor, Henry, greeted me on my cellphone line when I answered. He *never* called this late. His voice was anxious and direct, with hints of sadness and resignation.

"Karl, tonight we found Nancy outside your house in her nightgown. She was locked out of the house, wobbly, and drunk. I went back to our house to grab the spare house key you left with us. We opened the front door, got her back inside, and put her in bed. You really need to find a place for her NOW!" I thanked Henry for his kindness, attentiveness, and actions. I told him I would call Susan at once to ask her to find a bed for Nancy in an assisted living facility.

## Susan to the Rescue

Henry's phone call signaled the end of Nancy's solo living in our house. Henry was right. I needed to find a bed in an assisted living unit immediately. When I spoke with Susan early the next day, I explained the situation described by Henry. She was not surprised, understood the seriousness of the situation, and said she would immediately search for an available bed in one of the assisted living facilities she had already vetted for us.

By the close of business that first day, Susan found beds for Nancy at two assisted living facilities. We chose the one with less of an institutional feel. The next day, Susan was able to persuade Nancy that she needed to move out of the house, using the previous evening's sad episode of her being locked out of the house, drunk, and in nightclothes.

**PROFESSIONAL SOCIAL WORKER**

If you are the sole spouse or family member supporting a loved one with Korsakoff's, you may want to consider engaging a licensed professional social worker who specializes in eldercare. They know resources and can help you with supporting your loved one.

Within 48 hours of Henry's call to me, Nancy was admitted to a beautiful, assisted living facility, and she lives there to this day.

Nancy and I were fortunate to have found Susan. She was an experienced, credentialled social worker. Her retirement business centered on helping seniors and their families to find resources, even helping them with medical appointments, among other services. I never knew such resources existed until someone suggested this possibility to me. Susan was a godsend, as she helped me cope with the logistical demands of our situation over several years. Nancy liked her, and Susan was immensely helpful. After I left the house in April, Susan was our lifeline to take Nancy to medical and other key appointments. She was our angel, and she continues to support Nancy.

Within three days of Nancy's placement in the assisted living facility, I flew back to New England to retrieve furniture, clothes, jewelry, and other items from our home to take to Nancy's assisted living unit. Her own furniture replaced the spartan, but serviceable, pieces provided by the assisted living facility for her emergency admittance.

Nancy's small one-bedroom unit was now fully livable with her own belongings. Most importantly, Nancy was safe from herself and so was society. She was (and is) well-cared for with three meals, monitoring, and social programs.

# Chapter 21

## Third Neurological Evaluation

In early 2015, Susan accompanied Nancy back to the neurology center. A third neuropsychological evaluation was conducted solely because the assisted living facility staff and Susan thought they recognized improvements in Nancy's memory.[53]

The results of the third evaluation showed Nancy was still unaware of her memory challenges, and Dr. Jones' conclusions from this third test battery were unchanged from the second neurological evaluation. While showing some improvement in social measures (not surprising since she was now living in assisted living and not alone at home), Nancy significantly declined in the critical measures of processing speed, visual and verbal memory, and visual discrimination. Dr. Jones also concluded, despite about nine months of forced abstinence, it was unlikely Nancy would recover much (if any) memory. The report said Nancy was now vulnerable to other neurological conditions such as Alzheimer's Dementia in addition to her existing Korsakoff's Syndrome.[54]

Dr. Jones recommended that Nancy remain in assisted living with 24/7 supervision for her safety and to maintain sobriety. Because of the brain damage, her balance may be impaired, so the assisted living staff needed to monitor her. She also needed supervision on tasks requiring memory, finances, and medications.

---

**POWER OF ADDICTION**

The power of addiction cannot be underestimated. Dr. Grisel's book, Never Enough, will help you to better understand addiction.

---

This third evaluation underscored for me the devastation of alcoholism and dementia on a person's quality of life, relationships, finances, and more. I underestimated the power of addiction. I wish I had found Dr. Grisel's book, *Never Enough*, earlier to alert me to the challenges faced by substance abusers and their loved ones.[55] I also lacked the information and experience needed to understand how best to intervene and motivate alcoholics to take responsibility to move to sobriety.

I am still saddened by Nancy's decline from a weekend social drinker to an alcoholic with Korsakoff's Syndrome. Her slow but progressive decline was unchecked, and I did not see the seriousness of her addiction. This story may have had a happier ending if earlier interventions had led to Nancy's sobriety in time to prevent the onset of Korsakoff's, or if we had possessed the knowledge to act earlier on Nancy's early-stage Korsakoff's Syndrome symptoms.

In addition to now understanding the power of addiction, I see the pitfalls of rationalization where abnormal behavior is normalized. We become numb to actions and behaviors outside of acceptable bounds, and we make excuses or suppress what we know to be true. Perhaps I did not *want* to acknowledge her budding addiction in our codependent relationship.

What if I had been more aggressive in attempted interventions with Nancy when her friends and I first noted her alcohol abuse? What if I had sought professional guidance on living with alcoholics, joined Al-Anon, or explored our codependent relationship? Would we have helped alter the course of her alcoholism? I will be forever haunted by "what ifs."

# Chapter 22

# Moving Out/Moving On

Nancy's placement in the assisted living facility was a blessing for her and me, given her cognitive impairment and support needs. She was and is isolated from alcohol. With her placement, we had addressed yet another of the five recommendations made by the neurological team: providing Nancy with 24/7 support.

Her move now left our house vacant. As affirmed in her third neuropsychological assessment, Nancy's impairment was now irreversible. I was living in Florida and likely to remain, so we needed to either sell or rent the house. I had no interest in being a long-distance property owner, nor did I wish to pay Nancy for her half-ownership of the house or move back to New England. The decision to sell was easy. This decision necessitated preparing our house for its eventual sale.

## Move and Selling

In the second half of 2014, I made several trips to New England to move and store my belongings, deal with legal matters, and check on Nancy. During those visits, I rented two storage units where I transferred clothes, books, my furniture, and other items. More than forty-plus years of accumulated goods and memories needed disposition. I implemented a plan to clear out our remaining belongings through a combination of local donations and disposal, and later by shipping essential goods to Florida.

In 2015, I made four more trips back to our house. In addition to clearing out the house, Mary (our realtor and friend) performed a walk-through and prepared a punch list of items needing immediate attention to pass a buyer's home inspection. She found several items needing attention, especially for a buyer with an FHA/VA loan.

In the previous ten years, Nancy and I spent over $200,000 to install a new 30-year-guaranteed roof, repaved driveway, enhanced landscaping, new Pella wood-frame windows for the entire house, and we remodeled our two full baths and the half-bath, as well as the kitchen. Our retirement financial plan assured us of outright ownership of the house in 2016. With no mortgage, we planned to sail into our financially secure retirement. Although that plan was unattainable now, all the past home improvements would help us to sell the house quickly.

I brought back our remodeling contractor, Frank, to complete the home repairs and the final remodeling needs for the home sale. (You will meet Frank again in Chapter 27.) Painters refreshed our walls with neutral colors, and flooring contractors replaced carpets and refinished upstairs hardwood floors.

I was ruthless in clearing out our house. I had little time and no help. I stuck to my schedule and just kept moving. I maintained my workout routine to remain healthy and sane, arranged for dinners and happy hours with local friends, and worked part-time work for my regular employer who accommodated my need for personal leave during these challenging times.

## Reflection on What's Important

I was ready to move on. In the end, I shipped only a few possessions to Florida. Most objects had lost importance. When I worked in France for a year in the mid-1980s, I left the US with only two suitcases and one briefcase. That's all I needed. Having fewer possessions was somehow freeing, and now I felt similarly.

During my many trips in 2014 and 2015, I trucked useful items to Goodwill, Habitat for Humanity, and the Salvation Army. Many household goods no longer held any meaning to me, and I did not want to be burdened by them. The association of all these goods with our now-imploded marriage no doubt affected my affinity for these goods. But a load was lifted from my shoulders when I disposed of them.

Nancy had no more room in her small, assisted living unit. I also wanted to minimize the costs of shipping goods to Florida. I hired 1-800-GOT-JUNK to haul away five loads from the house and two loads from my storage units.

The house, the goods, and the upkeep were out of my life. Health, friendships, relationships with colleagues and others in my circle, and mental survival were more important.

At this stage of my life – at the time of this writing, now over nine years since my April flight to Florida – I reflected on my new priorities versus those that I had in my earlier adult years. I did not devote enough time to personal relationships. I spent too much time volunteering for political campaigns and participating in various government advisory committees and non-governmental organizations. I spent too much time working.

I once heard this phrase, and I wish I had heard it when I was 29 years old: "No one laid on their deathbed saying, 'I wish I could have worked one more day.'" *Why can't we see this when we are younger?* We are eager to prove our professional prowess, our commitment to be a martyr for the organization, and to receive accolades for our successes. Certainly, some of that is healthy, but I realize I overdid it. Accolades quickly fade in today's short-term focused corporate cultures of "*What did you do for me today?*" In the end, if you do not have relationships and your health, you have nothing.

By the time we moved, Nancy moved into assisted living in August 2014, and after the grind of living with Nancy's alcoholism and dementia, my depression had deepened. At age 64, my weight had dropped to 160 pounds, which is what I weighed as a scrawny eighteen-year-old entering college. I was now gaunt, tired, joyless, and sad. Unfortunately, the move to Florida to start a new life did not immediately remedy this state. Rebuilding my life was, and still is, arduous work requiring all the resiliency I can muster.

# Chapter 23

# Legal Matters

## Separation, Divorce, and Guardianship

When I flew to Florida in April 2014, I began my formal legal separation period from Nancy. State law required 365 days of not living under the same roof with your spouse and with total sexual abstinence from one another. Other legal milestones also loomed. We needed to engage legal counsel for the separation and divorce settlement negotiations and a later divorce filing. Because of Nancy's increasing cognitive impairment, we also needed to find a guardian for Nancy and then submit our formal filing with the Family Court for a guardianship appointment for Nancy.

The guardianship was necessary because Nancy's third neuropsychological evaluation confirmed her memory decline, the presence of Korsakoff's Syndrome, her lack of self-awareness of her memory challenges, and her drinking history. In addition, her neurological team recommended that a legal guardian should be appointed to assist with financial decisions, overseeing her assisted living arrangements, and overseeing the divorce settlement negotiations.

## Finding the Right Legal Counsel

Nancy and I initially engaged the wrong attorneys to negotiate our legal separation and divorce agreements given *our* circumstances and desired outcomes. Our divorce filing was not typical. It was not a case of domestic violence, financial irresponsibility, extramarital affairs, or unreconcilable differences. Ours was complicated by Nancy's Korsakoff's

**SELECTING YOUR ATTORNEYS**

Before signing engagement letters, I suggest you ask your prospective attorneys about their experience with clients who have dementia, especially with alcoholics and with Wernicke-Korsakoff's Syndrome. If you have already engaged with attorneys who do not grasp the crucial challenges of WKS in developing solutions in these unique situations, you may need to consider changes in your engagements.

Syndrome and alcohol-induced dementia. When engaging attorneys to assist with legal cases involving WKS and alcoholism, we learned it was important that our attorneys have experience and temperaments suited to address these uncommon health-related drivers.

My first attorney filed the separation agreement with the courts, but he made little progress with Nancy's attorney on the voluntary divorce settlement agreement. Nancy accepted the separation and divorce, and our attorneys knew we were not contesting the divorce. We did not have issues with equal division of property or other standard terms. However, Nancy's attorney simply dug in and refused to engage in negotiating the divorce settlement agreement. She rejected our first draft and said we should resubmit a revised draft, though she would not articulate her desired terms of the settlement agreement. No progress was made, and my attorney offered no ideas on how to break this stalemate.

After months of no progress and mounting legal bills, Nancy and I agreed the *status quo* was unacceptable for both the lack of progress and our individual steady cash outflows for legal fees *with no results.* We agreed that each of us would seek new legal representation.

I re-engaged an attorney who helped me a few years earlier when I wanted to learn about the state's divorce law and procedures. While her fees were higher than my first attorney, she knew me and understood our unique circumstances.

Nancy also switched to an experienced family law attorney who had also practiced in areas of guardianship. She understood this unique situation. Even better, we soon learned that both of our attorneys knew one another. They had a long-established professional relationship of mutual respect and an ability to work together to find solutions for their clients. Their ability to work together, and to recognize the unusual nature of our situation, made all the difference. Immediately, we made progress and soon completed the divorce settlement agreement.

---

**GUARDIANSHIP COUNSEL**

If your loved one has been diagnosed with Korsakoff's Syndrome, and if you need to establish court-appointed guardianship for them, you may need to engage a law firm to assist you with filing guardianship papers with the courts. You may also need to locate a person willing to serve as a guardian.

---

## Guardianship

While Nancy and I solved the issue of our individual legal representation, our uncontested divorce was not finalized until April 2016, in part because we needed to obtain a court-appointed guardian for Nancy. For that step, I engaged another local law firm with specific expertise in adult guardianship that could orchestrate the filing of the guardianship papers with the Family Court. This firm was experienced and respected, thus the Court efficiently managed the firm's filings.

We needed to identify a guardian for Nancy who would be named in our guardianship request filing. Our guardianship law firm found a local attorney with guardian experience who consented to be named as Nancy's guardian. We submitted her name in filings with the Family Court, and soon received the Court's decree appointing her as Nancy's guardian. The appointment of a guardian was a critical path step toward finalizing our divorce terms.

## Divorce Decree

Once the Family Court appointed Nancy's guardian, we filed our divorce papers (including our negotiated settlement agreement). Our hearing before the Family Court's magistrate was quickly scheduled. The divorce proceeding before the magistrate was brief and without any significant drama because the divorce was uncontested.

At the hearing, neither Nancy nor her appointed guardian were present. Nancy was represented by her attorney of record. The magistrate asked me perfunctory questions for which my attorney had briefed me earlier that morning. Satisfied with our filing and the signed voluntary divorce settlement agreement, the Family Court magistrate declared our divorce granted, the papers were signed, and I walked out of the county courthouse with the official declaration. It felt anti-climactic and was a sad day.

## Suggestion

I am not a practicing attorney nor formally studied in the law. However, I suggest to my readers that you should not hesitate to switch attorneys if they are ill-suited to meet your unique legal needs in the face of alcoholism and WKS. If we had first asked our prospective attorneys about their experiences with alcoholism, dementia, and guardianship, our legal experience would have been far smoother, more efficient, and cheaper.

# Part 5

## Rebuilding:
## Grief, Trauma, and Loyalty:
## 2016-2022

# Chapter 24

## Loss and Grief

Losing Nancy and our relationship was difficult to accept and occasionally waves of grief still wash over me. I have thought about Kubler-Ross' five stages of grief: Denial, Anger, Bargaining, Depression, and Acceptance.[56] While some contemporary observers and researchers have found little empirical evidence for these five stages of processing guilt, these stages held true for me, though not necessarily in that sequence. For me, Denial and Anger occurred simultaneously, though Anger simmered for years. My Bargaining stage was nonexistent because it was unclear to me with whom I would bargain. Depression – yes, check that box. I needed (and still need) professional mental health support. The black hole of depression still tugs on me from those ten-plus years of coping. Thankfully, three therapists helped me over the years.

As for Stage Five, Acceptance, I still have not accepted the loss. Yes, I understand it intellectually, but the underlying causes of Nancy's devotion to the bottle are still senseless to me. Obviously, Nancy needed something the bottle provided. I have acknowledged the outcome and the need to move on, but I have not accepted the tragedy of her alcoholism, her resultant Wernicke-Korsakoff's Syndrome, or the loss of our long-time relationship.

In my early years after moving to Florida, I knew that Nancy's assisted living residence was her destiny. I moved out physically in April 2014, but I continue to look for ways to move on mentally and emotionally. I continue to struggle to find genuine peace with the loss of our long-time relationship, and the clouds of sadness have not entirely dissipated. My therapists and I searched for effective therapies to help me accept my loss, so I could more fully embrace life and restore joy. As described in the next chapter, we increasingly viewed my sadness and inability to restore joy through the prism of trauma's impact.

# Chapter 25

# Recognizing and Treating Trauma

Before my ten-plus years' experience with Nancy's alcoholism and Korsakoff's Syndrome, I never thought that trauma could result from the cumulative effects of domestic life events. I always associated trauma with sudden, one-time exposure to violence, serious injuries, or domestic or sexual abuse. However, I learned it can occur from sustained, demanding, intense living over time coupled with significant emotional and mental challenges affecting one's ability to function in the modern world. It's not "just in your head" and it is not weakness or lack of discipline. It is chemistry.

## The World Viewed through a Veil

After our divorce was finalized in June 2016, and in developing a new relationship with a long-time friend and now partner, Kate, I made progress in rebuilding my life. Unfortunately, I often did not feel engaged in my new surroundings. Sometimes I still do not feel present. I feel as if I am an observer hovering over my day-to-day life unfolding on the planet. Putting New England behind me and receiving the divorce decree enhanced my attitude and energy levels, but I rarely experienced joy, and I often felt numb and joyless.

I had been in therapy with Colleen (my Florida therapist). I felt less depressed but still not anything close to my old self. I improved on Colleen's depression scale of Levels 1 to 10. I moved from Levels 2-3 (not good) to Levels 7-8 (better). After several therapy sessions discussing this continued malaise, Colleen and I came to the same conclusion. While I had not suffered sudden trauma from witnessing a murder or seeing an Army friend die in my arms, the extended mental burden of my ten-plus years of living with Nancy's alcoholism and dementia had taken a toll on me.

In those ten years, my brain chemistry changed due to chronic stress, with resulting elevated adrenaline and cortisol levels pulsating throughout my body. I was mentally and physically spent. Colleen and I wondered if one of the consequences of those ten years was PTSD – Post Traumatic Stress Disorder.

I read several books about trauma and PTSD (see Resources appendix of this book). Colleen and I then agreed I might benefit from a widely practiced therapy to treat PTSD called EMDR, or Eye Movement Desensitization and Reprocessing.

## Understanding Trauma and Brain Chemistry

Having a science background, I was especially drawn to Bessel van der Kolk's book, *The Body Keeps the Score*, which explains the physiological changes in the brain resulting from trauma.[57] His descriptions helped me to understand the sequence of reactions that sometimes resulted in my propensity to either totally shut down or lash out.

As Dr. van der Kolk points out, trauma produces physiological changes in our bodies, including the release of stress hormones that affect how we process information. He explains how traumatized patients are hypervigilant about threats and become disengaged in their daily lives. He reviews the history of medical and psychological insights gleaned from research in the mid-to-late-twentieth century, including brain imaging techniques developed in the early 1990s. The effects of trauma were clearly mapped in brain scans, and scientists were able to trace the chemical pathways, leading to a better understanding of the effects of trauma.

His book also suggests solutions. He describes treatment approaches to help PTSD patients to regain the ability to live full, engaged lives. As the body reacts to stress and trauma, the body adjusts its chemical sequence and changes the way you feel and react. Your behavior is substantially influenced by your chemistry. Your chemical sequences and resulting behaviors are repeated unless you interrupt or change the sequence.

To be clear, acknowledging the role of chemistry at work in your brain in no way absolves a person of their conscious ability to control their actions. People are still responsible for their actions, but by understanding the chemistry and behavioral responses, individuals can alter their behaviors and their engagement in life.

My copy of van der Kolk's book is full of notations. The insights I gleaned from his work have been life changing. Using his book to understand brain chemistry, I mapped my reactions to threats and their effects. I diagrammed my chain of reactions to events and demands that started during Nancy's growing alcoholism, the years of coping with her diminished cognitive state, and my residual stress after leaving New England. This recognition enabled me to better understand my triggers and responses (see Figure 2) which then helped

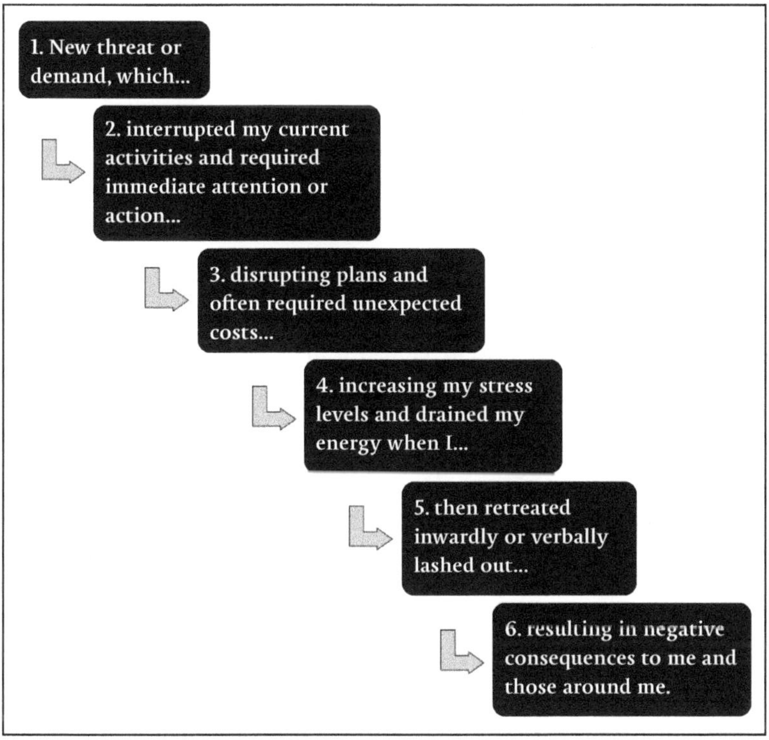


Figure 2. Author's Response Sequence to Trigger Events

Source: Author

me to modulate my responses. I could recognize the initiation of the default sequence and then interrupt the chain of events.

While understanding and interrupting the trigger sequence is certainly helpful, it is ideal if one can directly address the underlying triggers. Enter *Eye Movement Desensitization and Reprocessing therapy.*

## EMDR and Treatment of Trauma

Dr. van der Kolk described Eye Movement Desensitization and Reprocessing (EMDR) therapy, an established treatment for trauma. For more information about EMDR, I then read Dr. Francine Shapiro's book, *Getting Past Your Past*, which outlines the origin of EMDR, how it works, and the underlying reasons why it works.[58] She also offers simple techniques that one can use for self-help to cope with trauma.

By chance, Dr. Shapiro (a graduate student at the time) discovered the connection of eye movement to reduce a person's emotional disturbance. This discovery evolved into EMDR which, after validation studies, became a recognized treatment protocol to treat PTSD.

After I read both books, Colleen and I decided that EMDR might be helpful as I continued to struggle with depression and PTSD effects, which were threatening my relationship with Kate and my job. I struggled to contain frustrations and deep sadness.

While scientists have not yet mapped the exact neurological sequences in the brain that makes EMDR therapy effective, the result of applying this therapy is proven to enable patients to detach the emotion from a traumatic event, enabling the patient to heal and move forward. Patients do not forget the traumatic events, but after EMDR, they are able to view it as *an event* without an emotional charge.

As an accepted treatment method, mental health professionals can obtain certifications for EMDR's use with patients. I located several area therapists who were certified. I evaluated their credentials, experience, and their target client groups and then conducted phone interviews with my two leading candidates. I decided to pursue treatment with Stan.

In my first four sessions with Stan, we explored the events of my trauma. In EMDR, patients identify a traumatic "trigger" – ideally a specific event or circumstance – which becomes the "target" for the actual EMDR therapy. But my situation was not the typical sudden trauma from the battlefield, car crash, or abuse. It was complicated because my trauma was drawn out over ten-plus years. After four sessions, Stan and I settled on the image of Nancy's empty vodka bottle sitting on our kitchen counter.

In our fifth session, Stan applied EMDR therapy using our agreed-upon mental image of a bottle of Nancy's favorite vodka as the "trigger" image. At the conclusion of this fifth session, the bottle morphed from a memory that ignited the stress response to just a bottle.

How can that be? How can Nancy's bottle of vodka, which was a symbol of our dissolved marriage, become *just* a bottle? I acknowledge it seems like a bit of a stretch, but employing EMDR helped me to move on. Much of the anger evaporated, though some sadness remains due to the significance of that bottle. To this day, I cannot drink Nancy's favored brand of vodka, nor do I want to even see that brand's bottle. However, EMDR treatment helped to reduce the emotional charge (or the trigger) of what the bottle represented.

EMDR was one tool in my toolkit that I discovered with the help of my mental health professionals. While it has not ended my depression and the emotional charge of those ten-plus years, it helped to lessen the impact of my trauma.

## Moving Forward from Trauma, Loss, and Grief

Through EMDR therapy and psychotherapy, my ability to identify and modulate my reactions to threats and demands (Step 1 in Figure 2) empowered me to avert most of my automatic responses (Steps 5 and 6) with the resulting consequences (Step 6). EMDR reduced – though did not eliminate – the initiation of my default response. I became more social again and began to deepen my relationship with Kate. Nonetheless, I had lost my best friend to the bottle, and our planned future was dashed to pieces like the ship on the shoals. Despite EMDR therapy, I still felt some despair.

How could I shake this despair and move on in a way where I could restore a life filled with joy, love, and meaning? I worked through my day-to-day challenges and moved forward as best I could without complaint. I functioned proficiently in my job. I restored my workouts. I lived with Kate, a supportive woman who had been a long-time friend. She had her share of challenges with cancer, job loss, divorce, being a single mom, and being a leader in her professional field. Both of us held similar values, had attended similar types of schools, and had similar interests. She has been and is a wonderful part of my life.

She could sense that something was still missing even after my EMDR therapy and my continued therapy with Colleen. I was still detached and operating in some of my old patterns. I had not been able to quite shake the depression and my mood swings. I was not always the most pleasant person to be around, though I was progressing in my recovery. I had not really processed grief or accepted what had occurred back East.

I found another helpful resource in Christina Rasmussen's book, *Second Firsts: A Step-by-Step Guide to Life after Loss.*[59] She leads readers through a series of steps of recovery from trauma and loss based on her own experiences. Ms. Rasmussen found ways to move on after her husband succumbed to cancer. Her writing deeply engaged me. The depth of her grief from her loss, and the pathways she found to help her move on, resonated intimately with me. She described it as her Life Reentry Model. Her book, like those of van der Kolk and Schapiro, spoke to me. Like my copies of Shapiro and van der Kolk, my copy of her book is also filled with notations.

In *Second Firsts*, she spoke to the world in which I was living. She wrote about the three phases to a healthy recovery from a loss: exiting our old life, living in a gap between lives, and beginning to experiment with our new life. I can attest to these three phases. Like Dr. van der Kolk's book, she tells us that our brain chemistry changes from our trauma, our uncertainty, and our associated fears. Adrenaline pulses through our veins in our flight-or-fight response. Our world is uncertain and confusing, and we see threats everywhere. She, like I, constantly felt under siege.

Rasmussen's book reinforced Schapiro's and van der Kolk's books in helping me to understand how brain chemistry can be altered and why I was still reacting to the long-term demands from Nancy's alcoholism and Korsakoff's. No wonder I had been (and still was) worn out, edgy, and prone to immediate action with the attending physical and mental demands. I had no downtime, save for my periodic week-long caregiver respites. Understanding the underlying reasons for my reactions and feelings helped to calm me.

Her book illustrated a pathway for rebuilding a new life after trauma. She wrote that trauma can become a launching pad for your new life, but it requires active engagement and rethinking your life and how you live.[60] Rasmussen also cites lack of trust as a major hindrance to moving on – trust in other people (for me, a reaction to Nancy's betrayal) and trust in ourselves that we can rebuild our life.

The deepness of my mental exhaustion and emotional scars has slowed my rebuilding. However, the cited resources have been immensely helpful in restoring my optimism, gratitude and joy, and sociability.

## Restoration

I have not yet fully restored my attitude of being positive and joyful. On occasion, I still bemoan having my life upended, losing my best friend, and losing half of my assets as I entered retirement. The "perfectly planned" retirement that Nancy and I had built was sharply curtailed. But I still seek to remain positive. After moving from New England, I remained in contact with Katherine. I needed that touchpoint with her. Katherine knew me well, kept me honest, and implored me to be kind to myself. She underscored that I had done all I could for Nancy, had kept my job, took care of Mom with my sister, was healthy, and was thriving in a new relationship. Then Colleen, my Florida therapist, helped me to progress further.

Sometimes, I feel robbed of my best years. I planned well, and I had an excellent job with retirement only a couple of years away. The house would have been paid off, and we would have a decent retirement nest egg. Those plans vaporized. I wish I could report that I have fully moved on and am happy, but it is not the full truth. I have changed for the better in many ways – more humble, more tolerant, more understanding of others, kinder to myself, and more appreciative of my sister, Kate, and my friends.

My experience reinforced the need for me to tell my loved ones that I love them. I am grateful for what I have. I understand love better. The crucible that I survived made me stronger. I press on, seeking to rebound from adversity and my demons. I hope this chapter gives you some comfort that resources and treatments are available to help you move on from trauma.

# Chapter 26

# Loyalty

As a loyal husband, I sought to find solutions to help Nancy achieve abstinence which in turn was essential to any hope of restoring all or some of her cognitive capacity. Vocal friends said I was loyal to a fault, which might even be identified as codependency.

Can a spouse or partner, or even another family member or friend, be *too* loyal to their own detriment? In his thought- provoking book, *Loyalty: The Vexing Virtue*, author Eric Felton suggests that loyalty depends on both parties supporting one another.[61] Within Felton's framework, Nancy no longer supported our relationship, and I took loyalty too far, to my own detriment.

In this chapter, I examine loyalty because you may face decisions that test your bonds of loyalty. You may find the framework in this chapter useful in thinking through commitments, oaths, and future actions. I have not examined the body of literature on codependency but would suggest to my readers that they may want to augment their readings to include codependency.

We make imperfect choices, whether applied to our lives in general or specifically in the context of caring for both ourselves and our loved ones with Alcohol Use Disorder and WKS. *But indecision or lack of honesty with yourself and your loved ones may prolong an unhealthy and unsustainable relationship to the detriment of all parties.* In the context of alcoholism and Korsakoff's Syndrome, you may even miss opportunities to salvage the relationship and your loved one's future. Let's now explore loyalty.

## Scars and Loyalty

I was robbed of good years that can never be returned, and of course, Nancy changed her own life path. However, the feeling of being robbed is the *victim's view*, even though Nancy left me for the bottle. As an accountable adult, I should say: *I did not intervene soon enough in my own life, and I trapped myself in the cloak of loyalty and codependency.*

Perhaps I was lazy, or I desired even our flawed companionship, or I lacked the self-discipline to effectuate an earlier split with Nancy when she had continued drinking before her WKS diagnosis. In any event, it was *convenient* for me to stay with Nancy even when her alcohol abuse worsened, and she would not work to abstain. In retrospect, I rationalized her early behaviors, thinking, "*Oh, it's still only social drinking*," when deep down I knew she had a problem with alcohol. In the end, leaning on that rationalization proved detrimental to me and Nancy.[62]

After living with an alcoholic, you may need to make a personal decision about your own commitments when day-to-day life with an alcoholic loved one is no longer tolerable or healthy: *"Do I stay or not, and if I stay, on what terms?"*

*When do you call the question?* That is a highly personal decision. No one's situation is the same, and certainly, no one else can make that decision for you. I cannot advocate for a course of action for others, but for me, our wedding vows included "until death do us part," which was a serious commitment and responsibility. But when your equal partner indulges in reckless, self-serving behavior to *your* detriment, one might legitimately question marriage vows and loyalty between the two of you.

In the end, I tolerated Nancy's alcoholism for too long. Later, when it was clear Nancy had a disease beyond alcohol and there was no one else to help, I stayed because a friend helps a friend and I hoped we could salvage our marriage.

## What Is Loyalty?

I pondered the concept of loyalty over the last eight years or so, and I have reflected on the responsibilities of loyalty when living with an alcoholic. In his published lectures titled *The Philosophy of Loyalty*, Dr. Josiah Royce offered various definitions of loyalty. He said loyalty is not just an emotion because those who are loyal are committed to a cause that involves some submission of their natural desires.[63] If someone is loyal, they have a cause that they personally value. The loyal person believes in that value. The loyal person serves that cause without seeking personal advantage.

Royce also wrote that loyalty is founded on the belief that ties bind those who are loyal, and this in turn creates unity. Lovers would qualify as a cause because their love unifies them in something more than either of them alone. In my case, our love for one another was the cause, and the love and loyalty were reciprocated throughout the first half of our marriage.

Royce also wrote that there is a social element of loyalty: we are taught morality by our parents, churches, society, or other authoritative figures. However, in the end, individuals define duty, and it is a conscious decision.

## Questioning Loyalty

This discourse is important to my story and this book, and may be relevant to your life, too. When practicing loyalty, one may face an important question when loyalty is no longer reciprocated: *When is enough, enough?*

As for me, I held (and still hold) a deep-seated belief that true friendship and love involve implicit and explicit oaths, not unlike wedding vows or an oath to serve your country. If we are not loyal and if we do not value true friendship and sacrifice for friendship, then we are truly lone individuals who exist as disconnected human islands fending for ourselves. Without loyalty, friendship, and love, we would be alone. We could not count on anyone to help us when we were struggling. We would be alone in the Universe.

Without loyalty, we are profoundly alone, and we can trust no one. We would always be on the defensive and question the motives of others. We would see the world as a "zero-sum game" where one must fight for what is needed to survive. If I do not fight, someone else will take my portion. If there is no loyalty or deep, abiding friendship, then what do we have?

Loyalty provides part of the "nuclear glue" that supports personal relationships. My immediate family was small, consisting of only a few family members who were and are scattered across North America and Europe. As I developed in childhood and as an adult, the power of friendship and the agony of betrayal were central drivers in what I valued and desired. I did not and do not take friendships lightly. Friendships are to be treasured, nurtured, and honored. Maintaining these friendships requires active engagement.

For most of our lives together, Nancy and I had a deep friendship that sustained us and enabled each of us to grow and feel supported. We were not disconnected islands fending for ourselves. We were "in this to the end." We were a team. Our friendship became a source of unity and the object of our loyalty, using Royce's language.

## Breaking the Oath

If I had such a deep loyalty to true friendship, why did I leave Nancy in April 2014? The simple answer is that both the explicit and implicit oaths between us were broken. The oath to be there for the other devolved into a one-directional relationship or commitment where the other no longer acted to support those oaths.

For years, Nancy had the capacity to express her free will and to seek help to stop drinking, but she chose otherwise. She devolved from years of light-to-moderate social drinking to a full-fledged alcoholic. She disregarded the effects of her increased consumption on her well-being and mine, impacting her own ability to work. Out of loyalty, when I later realized she was impaired beyond alcoholism, I sought treatment for her. Unfortunately, her earlier choices still broke our oaths.

## Conflicting Loyalties

Royce discusses conflicting loyalties and how these are resolved. In my case, I had two conflicting loyalties, and there were four crucial decision points along the way in our lives together. The first loyalty was to our family unit, albeit it was only two people (that is, Nancy and me). The second loyalty was to the principle of taking personal responsibility and being accountable for one's actions. Both loyalties were called into question at *four* significant junctures in our relationship.

The first juncture was in 1989-1990, before Nancy's overseas postings, when I first recognized Nancy's increasing alcohol consumption and an inability to self-modulate her alcohol intake. It occurred at a business dinner at a downtown restaurant with an advisor to one of her clients, who was a well-respected, experienced leader in their field of practice. I was invited to join them. Later in the evening, while Nancy was using the restroom, our dinner guest told me that we should end the evening because Nancy was obviously drunk. I was mortified for Nancy and thanked our dinner guest for sharing her observation. Upon Nancy's return to our cozy table in this upscale restaurant, we said our goodbyes after settling our bill, and I whisked an unknowing Nancy off to our home.

She had embarrassed herself in front of a decision influencer of her future consulting work. I did not want to think about the consequences of Nancy's indiscretions that evening. At the time, I rationalized this night as a one-off occurrence, and the next day I only mildly noted to her the reasons the evening ended early. But the evening's events were startling enough to me that it registered as a "red flag." It was a troubling, out-of-character event. While I was unhappy about it, I made a conscious decision to forego a confrontation. In Royce's parlance, I had made a default, indecisive decision when faced with conflicting loyalties.

At the second juncture a few years later, I tried my first intervention with Nancy after her inebriated state at a business meeting (described in Chapter 3). I cited her performance to highlight her need to control her drinking. I shared with her the comments from fellow members about her state. I opted to try to support her to reduce her drinking in loyalty to our relationship. While I was beginning to suspect she was displaying alcoholic traits, I was unacquainted with alcoholism and was uncertain how to address these challenges. Hence, I did not fully pursue further actions to encourage her to reduce or end her alcohol consumption.

At the third juncture, I made another conscious decision in favor of loyalty. Having noticed her change of gait, memory challenges, and continued alcohol abuse, I initiated neurological healthcare actions to address her emerging symptoms of a medical condition beyond alcoholism. If I had not noticed her change of gait and apparent memory challenges, I would have left the relationship earlier. But when I noticed these disturbing behaviors, I concluded that a friend does not abandon a friend. She needed help, and she had no other family member who could help her.

At the fourth significant juncture of conflicting loyalties in April 2014, I finally resolved the conflict between the two loyalties (as described above). It was my tipping point. Nancy had disregarded all earlier attempts at intervention and had disregarded the unwritten oaths to support *us*. I knew I could no longer serve both loyalties and survive. I had to leave for self-preservation.

What was the result of my delays in "calling the question" and not facing the truth about Nancy's alcohol abuse? Both of us were disserved.

If Nancy abstained earlier, she may have been able to obtain value from alcohol addiction treatment *before* sliding into Korsakoff's Syndrome, and/or it may have resulted in a reversal of her cognitive impairment. But she did not control her alcohol consumption in her initial stages of alcohol abuse, and I did not call the question at the first three junctures. By not holding Nancy accountable to our relationship earlier (using Royce's parlance), we missed opportunities for Nancy to overcome her demons and to have altered the outcome of this sad progression of events. Also, I hurt myself by remaining too loyal.

## Honesty and Courage

My painful elaboration on the theme of loyalty here is quite deliberate. I implore my readers, who may be facing similar life-changing decisions: Think deeply about loyalty and honesty. Consider how the consequences of your decisions on care and your relationships may play out.

Having said that, let us acknowledge that we are still fallible human beings with imperfect knowledge. We are using only what is in our experiences and what we can learn from others to help guide us.

Twenty years ago, a longtime friend who was at least fifteen years older, wrote in her annual Christmas letter to Nancy and me – "It takes courage to be old."

I would add: *"It takes courage to be honest."*

Had I been more honest and truer to loyalties, had Nancy been more honest to me about her unhappiness, and had our neurological healthcare team been more transparent about the low probabilities of Nancy's addiction treatment success, then my life with Nancy and this story would have likely had a far different outcome – saving angst, time, financial resources, mental health, and perhaps even our relationship.

From these experiences, I suggest to my readers that you examine your loyalties and be driven by your conscience with honesty.

---

**HONESTY AND TRANSPARENCY**

A recurring theme in my experience is the need to be honest with yourself and to seek honest and transparent communications with your loved one, as well as with your health care providers, and addiction treatment professionals. In my situation, rationalization and deferral of tough decisions were detrimental to finding solutions and resulted in expending more resources with little to no benefit.

---

# Part 6

## Lessons and New Beginnings

Part Six is devoted to you, my readers. The lessons and questions in Part Six are derived directly from my experience with our health care and addiction treatment professionals from 2011 to 2015. In some cases, key topics were not discussed.

When a caregiver is the center of the maelstrom of pressing demands and elevated levels of stress, it is hard to identify your options or to think of the right questions. My hope is that my experiences and questions will aid you in making informed decisions for you and your loved one. I also offer my thoughts on how we as individuals move on from heartbreak and trauma.

The first chapter in Part 6 illustrates a challenge and offers a lesson in living with an alcoholic loved one.

# Chapter 27

## A Story: Look inside the Boot

Early one morning during a two-week stay to ready our house for sale, I sat at my makeshift desk upstairs in my home office in our vintage 1960s Cape Cod-style house in New England. Our contractor, Frank, who was also an ordained Protestant minister, beckoned me from the kitchen/living room level of the house.

"Karl, can you come down here for a minute, please? I need to show you something."

I set aside my client work, slightly annoyed with the interruption, and muttered to myself, *"Oh no, I wonder what Frank found now. What new repair work is needed?"* I lumbered down the freshly refinished oak staircase to our home's foyer.

At the bottom of the stairs, Frank held one insulated winter boot that he found in the coat closet as he cleared out its contents before working. He asked me to look inside the boot. I just stared motionless at the boot without uttering a sound.

Frank repeated his request, "Karl, can you please look inside the boot."

I glanced up at him and then once again down at the boot. My eyebrows furled. I was perplexed. I was expecting to hear about another new remodeling or repair need, but instead, I was facing a well-worn winter boot.

Once again, I glanced up at Frank with dismay and responded, "What? You want me to look inside the boot?"

Frank patiently repeated, "Yes, Karl, *look – in – the – boot*."

"Look in the boot? Really?" I asked.

Now exasperated, Frank repeated his request with a sigh. "Yes, Karl, *please* just look inside the boot."

So, I looked into the boot and beheld the sight of an empty brand-name vodka bottle. I looked back up at Frank, stunned at the incongruence of my expectations of more remodeling work *versus* what I now saw inside the boot.

I sighed and said, "I looked *everywhere* for her stashes, but I never thought to look in our winter boots."

Frank gently nodded his head and knowingly replied, "Alcoholics are very clever people."

# Chapter 28

# If You See Something, Say Something

## Friends Help Friends

In our post 9-11 world, we see placards on the walls of bustling train stations, and we hear disembodied voices on airport loudspeakers reminding us, *"If you see something, say something."* Travelers are asked to contact authorities about any suspicious behavior or unattended packages left near gates and boarding areas. This phrase also has relevance here.

Steve, a close friend of ours from the West Coast, often overnighted in our home when he traveled to New England for business. After a leisurely dinner, our evenings were normally accompanied by after-dinner wine, cognac, or cordials. I knew Steve was a night owl, though he drank in moderation. As the evenings wore on, Steve usually nursed his last drink for over an hour or two. He normally would retire after Nancy would finally end her alcohol-imbued ramblings from unrestrained drinking. Between the two of them, it was normally midnight or so before Nancy came to our bed and Steve went to the guest bedroom.

On these evenings, I was often in bed early for two reasons. My days began at 4:20 AM so I could begin my workout at our community fitness center at its 5:00 AM opening. If not driving to my workout, I would be in an early taxi heading to the airport for another business trip. More importantly, I could no longer bear the sight of Nancy being inebriated yet again late into the evening.

A few years ago, after I had moved to Florida, I was in Seattle on a business trip. Steve and I met for dinner at his favorite waterfront restaurant, Eliott's Oyster House. Before our halibut main course, we enjoyed Puget Sound oysters on-the-half-shell and Oysters Rockefeller. Steve soon confided that he had long noticed Nancy's alcohol excesses during his frequent visits with us. He said, "I hated to see Nancy in such a transformed state, from the self-confident, professional woman she once was to her drunken state." He lamented, "I wanted to tell you what I saw those late nights at your house, but I didn't know if I should say anything. Maybe I should have said something to you."

Before our dinner that night, Steve had not uttered a word to me about Nancy's readily apparent alcohol abuse. I long wondered what he thought during his many evenings at our home, but now I knew. I thanked him for sharing his observations with me, and I said, "I know it's hard as a friend to know what to say or when." I had been in similar positions with friends and close co-workers.

## But What Do You Say and How Can You Help?

The answer is quite simple but may be difficult to do. *Say something; anything.*

A simple observation would have been meaningful to me as the partner of an alcoholic: *"Karl, you know I care about you both. I've noticed Nancy seems to be drinking more, and it concerns me. I'm here for you both if I can be helpful."* No judgment; just caring and a desire to be supportive.

Steve's long-belated observations during our seafood dinner were still important. During our challenging years together, I sometimes questioned my perception of Nancy's situation and wondered if I had been too critical. Over time, I knew that was not the case, and that we had serious trouble. However, if Steve had said something when he

---

**FRIENDS AND FAMILY CAN BE HELPFUL**

When a friend or family member offers an observation of potential substance abuse or memory issue and it starts with love and caring, both parties benefit.

---

first observed Nancy's overconsumption, it would have been important validation. If a long-time friend was seeing what I was seeing, then I may have acted sooner to talk to Nancy about her drinking. But his belated comment that night during our fish dinner was still helpful.

My message is simply this: *saying something is an act of deep friendship and love.* Case in point: During a Friday after-work dinner three decades ago, a long-time family friend pointed out that I was sometimes cranky and ill-tempered before dinner. He asked if I ate a mid-afternoon snack while at work. I replied, "No, not really. Occasionally I might eat a cookie or apple, drink a Diet Coke, or eat something from the vending machine, but I don't make it a habit." Our friend suggested that I might want to regularly eat a granola bar, a piece of fruit, or something nutritious to keep my energy level stable in the afternoon. The following week, I followed our friend's advice, and it worked! I was no longer cranky and tired in the afternoon, and I was much better company.

My friend took a risk that I might be offended. To this day, I remember my friend's observation, and I often eat an afternoon snack because it still makes a difference in my late afternoon energy level and disposition. I am grateful that my friend took the opportunity to say something.

Offering your perspective to a friend is a minimal-risk offering *when it starts with care.* No one should be offended by such an observation. Please do not hesitate to tell a friend what you see. While difficult, your observation might significantly help your friend's situation.

# Chapter 29

# Making Decisions for Yourself and Your Loved One

## Lessons Learned the Hard Way

Life choices are rarely simple. Personal decision-making grows more complex as we age. Our choices as adults have potentially life-changing implications.

Even so, a particular choice might seem simple at first: for example, *"Should I rent this apartment, or should continue my search?"* But selecting an option typically involves considering many factors and tradeoffs. In this example, the decision to rent a specific apartment depends on the floorplan, parking availability, affordability, neighborhood conveniences, access to public transportation, types of appliances, and other features.

During my challenging years coping with Nancy's alcohol abuse and WKS, I kept a mental spreadsheet of the factors I needed to consider in make decisions for Nancy, me, or both of us. Sometimes, I even created simple tables or spreadsheets to list the factors.

On these mental or written lists, I used the questions and factors in this chapter to help me make many decisions about medical care, finances, and my own future.

After considering these questions, I needed to *balance* (or weigh) all these factors together to arrive at a decision. I cannot offer any suggested weightings for you as you balance the factors important to you; I do not know your circumstances. But these questions were central to my decision-making.

Beyond the factors I list below, readers may wish to review the

2020 book by Gail Weatherill on practical caregiving for dementia patients: *The Caregiver's Guide to Dementia: Practical Advice for Caring for Yourself and Your Loved One.*[64] At the end of each chapter, she asks the reader about their own status as a caregiver. I did not have this book as a resource at the time of our challenges, but her questions are spot-on to help caregivers ensure they are taking care of themselves, as well as making good choices for their loved ones with all forms of dementia.

One cautionary note: caregiving for loved ones who both abuse alcohol and have been diagnosed with WKS is unique. I recently found a self-published book written by David J. Steele, *Blackout: An Inside Look at Wernickes.*[65] His book is quite different than other commonly available self-help books or memoirs addressing dementia caregiving. Author David Steele was an alcoholic who was initially afflicted with Wernicke's Encephalopathy and then Korsakoff's Syndrome. I mention this book because it offers suggestions about treatments and caregiving from the patient's perspective.

## Decision Factors

You may find my list of questions below useful in your own decision-making. These are *not* ranked in order of priority.

1. **Loyalty and accountability** – What is the boundary between healthy loyalty and being too loyal? Are both of us holding to our oath of loyalty that we made to one another? Are my loved one's behaviors aligned with our commitments and standards to which we held each other accountable and to which we held ourselves accountable?

2. **Level of care needed** – Is my loved one receiving the level of care and/or quality of care that is appropriate to their condition? Is it the right care? Is an adjustment to the level of care needed?

3. **Self-preservation, survival, and self-care** – Are my own safety and self-preservation threatened or enhanced by supporting my

loved one? Can I physically, mentally, and spiritually survive the requirements placed upon me? Do I need help?

4. **Honesty and trustworthiness** – Is this person being honest with me? Are they telling me what they think I want to hear? Am I in turn honest with them?
5. **Friendship** – Would a real friend treat the other person the way they are treating me now? In answering this question, I decided that a "best friend" relationship implies loyalty, honesty, caring, and trust, while a casual friendship or acquaintanceship is less stable, with the tacit commitment of support and caring being less than a "best friend" relationship.
6. **Addictive behavior and potential interventions** – Are my loved one's behaviors consistent with those of a person with an addiction to alcohol, drugs, gambling, or other addictive disorders where professional interventions are needed?
7. **Codependency and Enabling** – Am I acting in a way that is supporting the other's well-being and my own well-being? Am I enabling my loved one to make self-destructive decisions, or to take actions that will cause to themselves or to me?
8. **Desire for companionship and continuance of the relationship** – How strongly do I still want to be in a relationship with this person? If I want to remain, is it because of love or loyalty? Am I simply avoiding change?
9. **Financial implications** – What are the financial implications of following a future course of action? Do I (or we) have the financial wherewithal to address a needed action or future circumstances? If not, what are the options and the probable outcomes?
10. **Employment responsibilities** – With my caregiving responsibilities, can I maintain my current level of commitment to my employer? If I am self-employed, can I provide proper service to my clients?

If I need to take personal or family care leave, does my employer offer such leave?

11. **Family responsibilities** – Have I fulfilled or am I fulfilling my duties of supporting the family? In my case, my immediate family was only Nancy and myself, but for a time, my sister and I also had responsibilities to ensure that our mother was cared for, safe, and secure. Hence, these commitments were part of balancing day-to-day decisions and plans to ensure I fulfilled agreed-upon responsibilities whether it be travel, phone calls with service providers, or finances at any point in time. If Nancy and I had had one or more offspring, their needs would have had to receive priority consideration, as well as in a situation where a parent lived under our roof.
12. **Legal responsibilities** – What are my responsibilities and accountabilities embodied in federal, state, and local laws, regulations, contracts, and other legal obligations? For example, our cars were registered in both of our names, so my attorney said that I could become a party to lawsuits if Nancy was responsible for a car crash resulting in injuries, deaths, or property damage.
13. **Mental state and capability** – Is my loved one capable of making decisions? Do they understand the implications of their actions? In my case with Nancy – was she capable of making changes on her own? Did she have enough self-awareness to do so?
14. **Our individual relationships to a Higher Power and our moral codes** – In considering an action, what are my responsibilities to a Higher Power in which I believe and with whom I have a relationship and/or to a religion or moral code to which I subscribe?
15. **Honest self-reflection** – Have I fulfilled my responsibilities to myself, to my loved one, and to the relationship? Where did I excel or fail? What is or has been my role? Was I supportive or indifferent? Did I act in a respectful, kind, and loving manner?

## For Your Consideration

I list these fifteen criteria for three reasons. First, negotiating pathways with loved ones and families through their alcoholism and alcohol-induced dementia is complicated. There are no cookie-cutter solutions to individual situations, just as there were no simple answers or solutions to my situation with Nancy. For your decision-making, you are the only one who can make an honest assessment of success, failure, regrets, luck, good fortune, or any other measures. But my fifteen questions were highly relevant to decisions I faced with Nancy's and my own care, and I submit they may be relevant to my reader's care decisions, too.

Second, you are not alone in the angst of balancing many factors as you decide on the proper courses of action in coping with your challenges of alcoholism and dementia with your loved one. It is not easy. Balancing competing needs and uncertainty is emotionally and mentally taxing.

Third, you may or may not agree with my criteria. For me, putting definitions around the factors going into my decisions was helpful. I submit that you will find it useful to borrow some of my fifteen factors, and customize the list to include your other factors that are meaningful to you and your circumstances.

# Chapter 30

# Five Important Information Gaps with Our Medical Team and Addiction Treatment Providers

While writing this book, I found five important information gaps at critical junctures that I did not recognize at the time I spoke with our medical, mental health, and addiction treatment professionals. In retrospect, the gaps outlined below were profoundly important. The answers to these questions would have likely steered us to take different actions, and we would have been better informed.

The gaps in patient-provider communications probably added two years and substantially greater costs for Nancy's treatments, care, and eventual placement in assisted living. Moreover, timely answers to these questions may have changed the course of our relationship, finances, and quality of life.

I have referenced these gaps in appropriate chapters throughout this book, but you may find these helpful to see them in one place.

## The Five Gaps

### Gap 1 – Probabilities of Successful Addiction Treatment for Patients with Korsakoff's Syndrome

Upon learning the results of Nancy's first neurological assessment, our neurological team told us that Nancy needed to stop drinking to potentially obtain a reversal of the effects of Korsakoff's. Our neurological team provided information about the general probabilities

**PROBABILITY THAT PATIENT IS CAPABLE OF ABSTIENCE**

1. Does [patient] possess enough self-awareness and capability with a diagnosis of Korsakoff's Syndrome to benefit from addiction treatment? With the patient's cognitive impairment and confabulation, can the patient abstain?
2. If not, are there other options?

of Korsakoff's patients' reversal of cognitive decline when they are abstinent and receive thiamine therapy. However, we did not receive guidance on the difficulty (or the improbability) of Nancy achieving abstinence given her level of impairment, lack of self-awareness of her situation, and confabulation. Even when she was placed under 24/7 monitoring for an extended period (as she was in residential addiction treatment, and later in intensive outpatient treatment), could she maintain abstinence on her own upon leaving treatment?

Unfortunately, after a year in three addiction treatment centers, we learned the answer to that question: *No*. The evaluation results told us she was impaired, that she lacked self- awareness of her situation, and she confabulated. How could addiction treatment have succeeded? Moreover, in the second assessment, we received the suggestion that she enter special residential treatment. Again, with her condition, how would that have been successful?

I should have asked the following two questions during our consultations with our neurological teams:

1. Did Nancy possess enough self-awareness to benefit from alcohol addiction treatment when she was diagnosed with a moderate level of Korsakoff's Syndrome with accompanying confabulation?
2. Is Nancy capable of acquiring the skills and awareness to remain abstinent after treatment ends?

I did not ask these questions, nor did our medical professionals address these issues. I simply accepted the neurological team's recommendations for Nancy's need to seek abstinence. It is disconcerting that no one directly told us then about the probable futility of sending Nancy to residential and intensive outpatient alcohol addiction treatment based on her incapacity to process the experience.

## Gap 2 – Referrals to Appropriate Addiction Treatment Facilities

In Nancy's first neuropsychological and neurological assessment, her medical team underscored her need to abstain from alcohol consumption and that she should seek treatment. However, in receiving the results of that first assessment, the team did not offer any referrals to specific qualified addiction treatment facilities with the competence to treat alcoholics with Korsakoff's Syndrome.

I was left on my own to find a suitable addiction treatment center. I should have asked the medical team for referrals to addiction treatment facilities which were equipped to effectively help patients achieve abstinence when they are afflicted with Korsakoff's Syndrome?

---

**REFERRALS TO APPROPRIATE ADDICTION TREATMENT CENTERS**

Ask your neurological healthcare providers: Do you have a list of addiction treatment centers that are equipped to effectively help patients with Korsakoff's to effectively work toward abstinence?

---

Only after receiving the results of the *second* neurological evaluation did our neurological team suggest one potential center in the Southern US (though the costs exceeded even the $35,000 per month of our local residential treatment center). I later found other expensive, out-of-state centers that were equipped to accept patients with Alcohol Use Disorder with WKS. But I did not have this information at the time of the neurological team's initial recommendations that Nancy should seek addiction treatment, and sending her to residential treatment after the second assessment would have been even more futile with her level of impairment, lack of self- awareness, and confabulating.

## Gap 3 – Successes in Treating Alcoholics with Korsakoff's Syndrome

Earlier, I noted that the first two addiction treatment facilities I contacted refused to accept Nancy solely because she had Korsakoff's Syndrome. In retrospect, these two rejections should have been a red flag or an alert to me: *Why did they establish a policy of not accepting Korsakoff's Syndrome into treatment?*

Surely, they either had earlier experience and/or medical knowledge that patients with Korsakoff's Syndrome would not or could not be successfully treated because they lack the capability to learn from treatment approaches.

I was so intensely focused on finding a treatment center that I did not ask these questions. These treatment centers did not offer any explanation beyond stating their policy.

If I were faced again with this situation, I would direct these eight questions to prospective addiction treatment centers (see sidebar). These questions focus on probabilities of success in treating patients with Korsakoff's.

---

**QUESTIONS FOR ADDICTION TREATMENT CENTERS**

1. Do you accept clients with Korsakoff's Syndrome?
2. If not, why don't you accept patients with Korsakoff's Syndrome?
3. If you accept patients with Korsakoff's, what is the probability of success that they will remain abstinent after leaving the treatment program?
4. Are patients with Korsakoff's capable of benefiting from alcohol addiction treatment? Can you ascertain those who would benefit from treatment and those unlikely to benefit?
5. What are the treatment options for achieving and maintaining abstinence in patients with Korsakoff's?
6. Based on your experiences with clients who had Korsakoff's, how long do they need to be under your direct care to remain sober after leaving your care?
7. What Vitamin B therapies would you recommend? What are your protocols? How do you monitor effectiveness? Do you work with the patient's neurological team?
8. Do you have evidence of treatment effectiveness in moving patients with Korsakoff's to abstinence?

---

Had I known to ask addiction treatment centers these eight specific questions after the first diagnosis by Drs. Jones and Smith at the medical center, the trajectory of Nancy's treatment could have been more effective. Or we could have acted sooner to place Nancy in assisted living or other monitored living setting with enforced abstinence.

## GAP 4 – VITAMIN B THERAPY

While writing this book, I learned that Korsakoff's patients fare better when an integrated medical team monitors the patient and approaches treatment holistically, including Vitamin B therapy with psychological assistance.

---

**VITAMIN B THERAPIES**

Ask your medical team to clarify their prescriptions for Vitamin B therapies:

1. If Vitamin B12 is being prescribed, what is the diagnosed condition?
2. If Vitamin B1 is being prescribed, what is the diagnosed condition?
3. In prescribing thiamine therapy, have you considered the patient's genetic disposition and her body's receptivity to absorb thiamine? What will be the most effective delivery mechanism?
4. If the effectiveness of Vitamin B therapies hinge on a patient's abstinence, and if the patient is not abstaining, should Vitamin B therapies be continued?

---

Nancy initially received Vitamin B12 therapies (injections and oral) from her first neurologist, though he did not name the specific condition for which Vitamin B12 was being prescribed beyond "mild cognitive impairment." (There are numerous conditions associated with alcohol-induced dementia.)

Nancy's second neurologist prescribed Vitamin B1 (thiamine) therapy for her WKS diagnosis.

The scientific literature demonstrates that the effectiveness of Vitamin B delivery methods varies by the individual based on genetic disposition, the extent of neurotoxicity from alcohol, the type of impairment, and more. It is also clear from the literature that the patient must cease alcohol consumption for therapies to be effective.

In Nancy's case, I should have asked our medical treatment providers the following four questions:

1. In prescribing thiamine therapy, have you considered Nancy's genetic disposition and her body's receptivity to absorb thiamine? What will be the most effective delivery mechanism?
2. If the effectiveness of Vitamin B therapy hinges on a patient's abstinence, and if the patient is not abstaining, should Vitamin B therapies be continued?
3. If Vitamin B12 is being prescribed, what is the diagnosed condition?
4. If Vitamin B1 is being prescribed, what is the diagnosed condition?

Based upon my experience, it is important to understand the Vitamin B therapy being used with your loved one.

## Gap 5 – Potential Direct and Indirect Effects of Menopause and Surgical Histories

Our medical and addiction treatment team did not ask us about the timing of Nancy's menopause, or her surgical histories related to female reproductive organs. The information gleaned from these discussions should have been factored into assessments and treatment plans – medical, mental health, and addiction treatments. The ultimate out-

**PERIMENOPAUSE AND MENOPAUSE CONSIDERATIONS IN ASSESSMENT AND TREATMENT**

Ask your medical, mental health, and addiction treatment professionals to consider the potential effects of perimenopause and menopause in their diagnosis and treatment plans. While I suggest it is better to address these factors at the outset of your consultations, you may still want to interject these considerations even if you are already engaged with these professionals.

comes may or may not have been different, though it's possible.

I suggest you add the following talking points for discussions with your medical, psychological, and addiction treatment teams:

1. Ask your medical and mental health teams to consider the timing of your loved one's menopause and the potential impacts of that timing on both heightened risks of dementia and alcohol abuse.
2. Ask your addiction treatment professionals to consider your loved one's menopausal experiences, and especially if they have experienced depression and anxiety that may have contributed to her alcohol abuse.
3. Ask your medical, mental health, and addiction treatment professionals to consider your loved one's surgical history as they develop diagnostic and treatment plans.

## Medical Challenges

The medical community continues to build a knowledge base about Wernicke-Korsakoff's Syndrome. For example, science is beginning to find genetic markers that may facilitate Vitamin B therapies. Hopefully, science can find dose-response thresholds for Vitamin B therapies beyond those available when we needed them. Future medical research may document better probabilities of the effectiveness of various treatment protocols.

It would be life-changing, too, if science could develop a medicine to alter brain chemistry to eliminate or reduce an alcoholic's craving.[66]

In addition, is it possible that researchers could find standardized indices for early diagnosis of Korsakoff's Syndrome? For example, Butters and Cermak noted studies showing that Korsakoff's patients appear to have reduced capabilities to discern odors.[67] Could a simple screening tool be developed for medical professionals that would enable doctors to make earlier referrals that could improve success rates for the reversal of cognitive impairments from earlier stages of Korsakoff's?

I am grateful for the diagnoses made by our neurological team, so we knew that Nancy's impairment extended beyond alcoholism. However, with Nancy's incapacity to alter her alcoholic behavior due to Korsakoff's Syndrome, it seemed to me that much of the time and resources spent – as well as the emotional drain – were wasted because this question of her capacity to change was not considered or discussed.

Ideally, I would have asked all these questions and more, but when you are in the middle of caregiving and coping, you cannot always see other options. I hope this chapter raises awareness among my readers of the need for robust patient and family communications with their medical and addiction treatment teams.

# Chapter 31

## Coping with the Demands of Caregiving

Christina Rasmussen, Bessel van der Kolk, Francine Shapiro, and others have written eloquently about techniques for moving on from trauma. This book is no substitute for their extensive guidance and the professional mental health care that is accessible today.

For guidance on how to move on beyond trauma, I found Rasmussen's Life Reentry approach to be especially useful. She writes that when we seek to move on, we are forced to change but we must begin with our existing body and mind and retrain ourselves.[68] No wonder personal growth and change are so hard! But in her writings, I found she has done us all a great service in laying out the steps on how to achieve such growth.

Bessel van der Kolk writes that when we make changes that become part of our lives, these changes alter our brain chemistry for the better. After the challenging work of change, we become rewired to maintain our momentum in personal growth.

### How Do We Move On?

In addition to working through Rasmussen's Life Reentry steps in recovering from the trauma of living with Nancy's alcoholism and Korsakoff's, I drew upon the books of Shapiro, van der Kolk, and others. I extracted several coping and change-management techniques that facilitated my growth and recovery; some were easier to adopt than others.

From their suggestions and my own experience, I found the following seven coping actions to be the most helpful to me. Perhaps you will find these useful in supporting your coping and change management skills, too.

1. **"Just five minutes"** – I used this catchphrase in two circumstances: when I needed to begin a task or phone call I dreaded; and, when I was so stressed by care demands that I felt panicked. I then simply began the task and gave myself five minutes to focus on one small doable task. After five minutes, I was free to move on to something else, but I still felt like I accomplished one goal. Moreover, I found that devoting a few minutes to one task often led to spending more time on that task, or I might even finish the entire task. Often this mind trick enabled me to clear my head of all the incoming missiles and freed me to work well beyond the set time and accomplish even more.
2. **Reach out for help and renew your support network** – I could not have survived my challenging years without the support of close friends and supportive co-workers. Friends and other people in your circles will want to be helpful, but they may not know how to help. You can help them to help you. Contact your best friends and ask them to help you with a few important tasks or invite them for coffee if you need to talk. My advice: reach out and fight the social isolation that accompanies alcoholism and Korsakoff's Syndrome in the family.
3. **Define what will give you peace, and take respite breaks** – In my dementia support group, and in two books, *The 36-Hour Day* and *The Caregiver's Guide to Dementia*, caregivers are cautioned about the need to take care of themselves. I was told that caregivers may die before their loved ones because of the physical and mental toll it takes on caregivers. I found escape valves through periods of respite where I could let down my guard. I periodically took three to seven days to travel out of town, seeking sunshine or walking opportunities, or to simply visit friends. I nourished my body and

my soul without guilt. Sometimes, my break was only a noontime walk in our neighborhood to feel the cool autumn breeze and the sun in my eyes. A respite might be reading an enjoyable book by your favorite author or a coffee break at your local coffee shop. It might be a couple of days at your favorite bed and breakfast or resort.

4. **Understand your triggers, and don't be afraid to seek professional mental healthcare professionals** – I discovered over time that I needed to understand the reasons behind my reactions to Nancy and other life events, including time during my recovery when I began living with Kate. The stresses resulting from the demands of being a caregiver were substantial and resulted in changes in my brain chemistry. I needed to understand my triggers, emotions, and "baggage" to cope with and, later, shift my brain chemistry to a more normal state.

   Bessel van der Kolk's and Francine Schapiro's books helped me, but my mental health professionals were my saviors. I needed their dispassionate, third-party objectivity and professional training to help me acknowledge my strengths and weaknesses and what I might do to encourage those strengths and address the weaknesses. Growing up, seeking mental health support had a stigma attached to it. Going to a therapist was something you hid. Thankfully, obtaining mental health support is now more socially accepted. My three mental healthcare providers gave me unvarnished perspectives to help me understand what I accomplished or needed to undertake and how to value myself. They helped me cope and repair parts of my life.

5. **Find resources to whom you can off-load some tasks** – In addition to your friends and family, you might want to identify needs and tasks that you can off-load to volunteers or professional service providers. In my case, I found Susan, our private eldercare social worker who specialized in helping families with finding resources, going with loved ones to medical appointments, and

more. I suggest you periodically list all the tasks that you need to complete and think about whom you might engage to undertake at least one or more tasks for you.

6. **Be kind to yourself** – While related to No. 3 above (giving yourself respite time), this item is related *to managing your expectations*. What we do as caregivers is physically, mentally, and emotionally draining. As a Type-A personality, it was easy for me to feel inadequate and that I could always do more. My two therapists helped me see that I was doing the right things and was coping remarkedly well. Initially, I could not see that, but they could. They, in turn, encouraged me to be kind to myself. Acknowledge you are doing the best you can under challenging circumstances and that you are worthy of goodness for a healthy and successful existence.
7. **Be your own and your loved one's advocate** – When I grew up, we saw "the family doctor" when we needed medical care, and we stayed with their practice until they passed away or we moved. We did not question his medical opinions. Fortunately, questioning a diagnosis or treatment plans – or seeking second opinions – are now more accepted, and for good reasons. No one is infallible,

---

**COPING SUGGESTIONS**

- For unpleasant or difficult tasks, say to yourself, "Just spend 5 minutes" to get started.
- Reach out for help and renew your support network.
- Define what will provide you with peace, and take respite breaks.
- Understand your "triggers" for anxiety and frustration, so you can better manage your communications and decisions.
- Find resources that will allow you to off-load tasks.
- Be kind to yourself.
- Be your loved one's (and your own) advocate.

In addition:

- Smile even if you don't feel like it.
- Be grateful for what you have.

---

and all of us have filters. You may need to seek second opinions and bring other professionals into your healthcare and/or addiction treatment teams to ensure you have the best possible positive health outcome for your loved one. My dementia support group was helpful since the discussion stimulated my thinking about alternative views and options. Most importantly, trust the voice within you, ask questions, and explore options with your healthcare providers.

## Life Lessons

In addition to my first-hand experiences and lessons with alcoholism, alcohol-related cognitive impairment, and dementia with related diagnosis and treatment, I also learned important life lessons during this difficult journey. I became more resilient, and I try to live my life with more gratitude, tolerance, humbleness, and kindness. I express my love and friendship to those I love and those who are my closest family and friends. I do not wait to say it. I strive to say it every day as if it is my or their last days on Earth.

Based on an idea from my therapist, Colleen, I wear a thin rubber wristband that I customized through an online supplier. The words "Be Grateful" and "Be Kind" are embedded in the band. I wear it 24/7 as my constant reminder to live this way. Also, when I feel agitated or frustrated and ready to make a rash statement, I gently snap the band as a reminder to pause.

I have methodically rebuilt my life and hopefully also enhanced the lives of people around me. The challenges of those years with Nancy made me a better person and showed me it is critical to reach out for help. None of us can do it all alone.

I am especially grateful for the gifts of love, kindness, and support through the years from my parents, my sister Beth, professional caregivers, incredible friends, and supportive co- workers. I am now especially grateful to Kate for her love and support. I do not know if she really bargained for this bundle of angst, baggage, and uncertainty, but we were longtime friends and each saw in the other honesty, kindness, strength, humanity, and the capacity for love.

While my journey continues and I still experience occasional lapses of deep sadness and sometimes residual anger, the EMDR treatment reduced much of the negative emotion. Occasionally, I am still short-tempered and impatient, but gradually my drivers of gratefulness, humbleness, and tolerance are increasing.

## The Mere Act of Smiling

Based on modern science, we now know that even if you do not want to smile, the mere act of making yourself smile will alter your brain chemistry in positive ways. **So, smile.** It is sometimes amazing to me how just a tiny smile will shift my mood and inner dialogue. Getting up from your chair or desk and moving or walking, helping someone, or undertaking a new task will also help you to feel better.

I am not advocating that you behave unauthentically. I simply suggest that you apply these suggested actions to help you along on your own journey of recovery. This is easier said than done. I am still young enough as I author this book to desire to evolve and persevere. I can choose to stay wounded and to succumb to depression and joylessness, or I can continue to strive for joy. I choose the latter, and my wish for you is that you can also do so.

# Chapter 32

## Key Takeaways

As I close out this book, I offer the following quick review of the key takeaways that, if followed, could change the course of your life and the lives of your loved one and your family:

**1. Ask questions of your medical and mental health providers and addiction treatment professionals.**

Why are they performing planned tests? What are the prescribed medications or treatments and why are they indicated for your loved one's condition? What have been their experiences with WKS patients seeking alcohol addiction treatment? Seek second opinions if you are not satisfied with their answers. While simple cognitive impairment can be initially identified with a basic in-office exam and a few questions, diagnosing WKS requires more specialized testing.

**2. Look for early signs of alcoholism and Wernicke-Korsakoff's Syndrome.**

Learn the early signs of alcohol abuse and WKS. The earlier your loved one is diagnosed with WKS and looks for medical and addiction treatment, the better the chances of reducing their cognitive impairment. Also, the sooner a loved one with Alcohol Use Disorder can find their way to abstinence, the sooner they reduce their risk for developing WKS. Acting early could be critical in potentially reversing some or all cognitive impairment of WKS. *Time is of the essence.* See the next key point.

**3. Be honest with yourself and your loved one.**

Rationalizing alcohol misuse behaviors or the early signs of WKS will only delay treatment that could change the course of your lives. Recognizing and addressing changes may save years of stress, living challenges, and significant dollar outlays. *Please do not rationalize abnormal behaviors or delay in seeking professional help.*

**4. Take care of yourself, and seek help to spread your burden.**

If you are a spouse, partner, or caregiver of a loved one who is an alcoholic and/or who has WKS, it is essential that you support your own physical and mental health. If your mental or physical health declines, both you and your loved one will be at risk. If you need help, ask for it from friends, support organizations, or even private elder-care social workers. If you feel overwhelmed and/or depressed, seek out support from mental health professionals.

**5. Become informed.**

While readers will find significant literature and resources on more frequently diagnosed dementias and cognitive impairments other than WKS, you may want to consult the resources I have listed in the appendix. For alcohol abuse, I can think of no better starting points than Alcoholics Anonymous, Al-Anon for families, and addiction treatment professionals. I had no experience with alcoholism, and I should have sought more help earlier in our journey.

# Chapter 33

# Love and Hope

Without hope, loyalty, and friendship, our lives can feel empty at best, and desperate and depressing at worst. I held out hope that the *next* attempt at alcohol addiction treatment would be *the key* to reversing Nancy's path. As a loyal partner with hope and persistence, I could not have lived with myself to turn away from helping Nancy once we learned of her alcoholism and the Korsakoff's complication.

## Love and Hope

Nancy and I were originally committed to our relationship and were best friends. We were in love up to the point where Nancy's alcohol craving overrode her love of herself, others, and our own love and relationship. We strove to create a household of support and love, which included our close friends, their children, and fellow "orphans" who were physically distant from their families. We had been a "safe house" on our block for latch-key school children in the neighborhood. Love for each other and love for our fellow sojourners in this life were essential parts of our lives.

For me, it was the love, friendship, and loyalty that drove me to give my all to help Nancy slay her demons so she could return from her alcohol-imbued world back to *our* world together.

I wish for Nancy that she has found a place of peace, and continues to receive quality care.

## Helping Each Other

Humans are fallible; we excel at some things – being a great parent, achieving a great accomplishment in our work life, or helping others thrive from our efforts to support them. We can fail miserably, too, in what we undertake due to ego, ignorance, self-importance, or expediency.

We all have challenges – financial, familial, educational, or emotional – but most of us want to thrive and help our communities, friends, and our loved ones. Sharing knowledge and experiences can help us all.

I had *no* roadmap for coping with Nancy's alcohol abuse and Korsakoff's Syndrome when my journey with her started. I offer my experiences, resources, and suggestions to help you plan and support your loved one. This book cannot and does not take the place of professional medical, mental health, addiction treatment, or legal guidance, but I hope it provides you with ideas and solace in knowing you are not alone in facing the challenges of alcohol abuse with Korsakoff's Syndrome.

I wish you well on your journey. May you take care of yourself and your loved ones, and may they overcome their demons with your support. May they reemerge as the loving partner or family member you knew and continue to love.

# Endnotes

1 - Sadly, I recently learned that Joe's wife died of liver failure after having renewed her alcohol abuse.

2 - Sanvvisen, Arantza et al. Long-term mortality of patients with an alcohol-related Wernicke-Korsakoff Syndrome. Alcohol and Alcoholism, Volume 52, Issue 4, July 2017, pp. 466-471. https://doi.org/10.1093/alcalc/agx013

3 - Michael D. Kopelman, Allan D. Thomson, Irene Guerrini, E. Jane Marshall. The Korsakoff Syndrome: Clinical Aspects, Psychology and Treatment. Alcohol and Alcoholism, Volume 44, Issue 2, March-April 2009, Pages 148– 154.

4 - SAMHSA, Center for Behavioral Health Statistics and Quality. 2019 National Survey on Drug Use and Health. Table 5.4A – Alcohol Use Disorder in Past Year among Persons Aged 12 or Older, by Age Group and Demographic Characteristics: Numbers in Thousands, 2018 and 2019. https://www.samhsa.gov/data/sites/default/files/reports/rpt29394/NSDUHDetailedTabs2019/NSDUHDetailedTabs2019.htm (Accessed December 8, 2020.)

*and*

SAMHSA, Center for Behavioral Health Statistics and Quality. 2019 National Survey on Drug Use and Health. Table 5.4B – Alcohol Use Disorder in Past Year among Persons Aged 12 or Older, by Age Group and Demographic Characteristics: Percentages, 2018 and 2019. https://www.samhsa.gov/data/sites/default/files/reports/rpt29394/NSDUHDetailedTabs2019/NSDUHDetailedTabs2019.htm (Accessed December 8, 2020.)

5 - Our experience focused on Korsakoff's Syndrome (KS), defined as a long-term (chronic) memory disorder. Some, but not all, patients affected by Korsakoff's Syndrome are first afflicted with Wernicke's encephalopathy (WE), which is a sudden and severe (acute) brain disorder. Both can be life-threatening if left untreated. For an excellent brief description of WKS, please see: Cleveland Clinic, Wernicke-Korsakoff's Syndrome. https://my. clevelandclinic.org/health/diseases/22687-wernicke-korsakoff-syndrome

6 - Nicolos J.M. Arts et al, Korsakoff's Syndrome: a critical review. Neuropsychiatric Disease and Treatment. 2017: 13, pp 2875-2890.

7 - According to the National Institute on Alcohol Abuse and Alcoholism (NIAAA), a standard drink contains around 14 grams (0.6 ounces) of pure alcohol. In the U.S., this can generally be found in 12 ounces of beer, or one bottle at 5% ABV; 8 ounces of malt liquor at 7% ABV; 5 ounces of wine at 12%

ABV; 1.5 ounces of hard liquor, or one shot, at 40% ABV; 8-9 ounces of malt liquor at 7% ABV. Source: https://www.alcohol.org/statistics-information/abv/

8 - "According to the "Dietary Guidelines for Americans 2020-2025," U.S. Department of Health and Human Services and U.S. Department of Agriculture, adults of legal drinking age can choose not to drink or to drink in moderation by limiting intake to 2 drinks or less in a day for men and 1 drink or less in a day for women, when alcohol is consumed. Drinking less is better for health than drinking more. NIAAA defines heavy drinking as follows: For men, consuming more than 4 drinks on any day or more than 14 drinks per week; and for women, consuming more than 3 drinks on any day or more than 7 drinks per week. Source: https://www.niaaa.nih.gov/alcohol-health/overview-alcohol-consumption/moderate-binge-drinking#:~:text=NIAAA%20defines%20heavy%20drinking%20as%20follows%3A%20For%20men%2C,day%20or%20more%20than%207%20drinks%20per%20week

9 - Kerry Egan, On Living. New York, New York. Riverhead Books. 2016.

10 - Grisel, Judith. Never Enough: The Neuroscience and Experience of Addiction. London, UK. Scribe Publications. 2019, pp. 80-102.

11 - Recently I learned that even drinking non-alcoholic beer and wine can be a trigger event for an alcoholic, leading to intense desires to imbibe. Hence, this naïve and well-meaning agreement undermined the environment I sought to create to support Nancy's purported abstinence.

12 - Additional signs and symptoms of WKS may include visual disturbances (including double vision, abnormal eye movements, eyelid drooping) and mental confusion (including memory loss and inability to form new memories). Note: WKS patients are often alert and possess good social skills.

13 - See also: Lindsay Leatherdale, Korsakoff's or Wernicke Korsakoff's Syndrome Explained. Is it Alcohol-induced Dementia: Wernicke-Korsakoff's Signs, Symptoms, Causes, Treatment, Stages of Tests All Covered. IMB Publishing, 2013.

14 - It is interesting to note that neither Dr. Jones nor later Dr. Edwards, mentioned Wernicke encephalopathy which often, but not always, precedes Korsakoff's Syndrome.

15 - For readers who wish to understand the mechanism of Wernicke-Korsakoff's Syndrome, a helpful review is in: Abin Chandra Kumer et al, Review of thiamine deficiency disorders: Wernicke encephalopathy and Korsakoff's psychosis, Journal Basic Clinical Pharmacology, 2019, Vol. 30, Number 2, pp. 153-162.

16 - About 25% of patients fully or mostly recover cognition, 50% have partial recovery, and 25% have no recovery.

17 - See: https://en.wikipedia.org/wiki/This_Is_Your_Brain_on_Drugs

18 - Mace, Nancy L. and Rabins, Peter V. The 36-Hour Day: A Family Guide to Caring for People Who Have Alzheimer Disease, Other Dementias, and Memory Loss. Baltimore, MD. Johns Hopkins University Press. 6th Edition. 2017.

19 - Weatherill, Gail. The Caregiver's Guide to Dementia: Practical Advice for Caring for Yourself and Your Loved One. Emeryville, CA. Rockridge Press. 2020.

20 - Harrison, Thomas F. and Forester, Brent P. The Complete Family Guide to Dementia. New York, NY. Guilford Press. 2022.

21 - In the Bibliography and Resources section, you will find reference material that I found more recently.

22 - Steele, David J. Blackout: A Look Inside Wernickes. Self-published. 2011. (ISBN: 978-1=105-04395-6).

23 - Recently, I learned from a therapist that such a situation, where an individual with alcohol abuse disorder drinks non-alcoholic wine, may constitute a "trigger event." In retrospect, we should have avoided the consumption of non-alcoholic wine and beer, as these activities may have reinforced Nancy's desire to drink her favorite alcoholic beverages. For more information, readers may wish to read: Samuel Asensio et al, "What is the "Trigger" of Addiction?" in Frontiers of Behavioral Neuroscience. April 21, 2020; 14: 54. Doi: 10.3389/fnbeh.2020.00054.

24 - Our neurological team had explained to us that we all have a "cognitive reserve" of our innate cognitive capacity. Think of this reserve like a savings account. We can sustain some level of "withdrawals" on that reserve, but in the case of cognitive reserves, the withdrawals consist of alcohol abuse, head injuries, and drugs (to name a few). We can make some withdrawals and still maintain our innate cognitive capabilities. But that reserve can be exhausted. In Nancy's case, these withdrawals from her cognitive reserve came from excessive alcohol consumption. Unchecked withdrawals can lead to memory loss and potential dementia. A summary of cognitive research can be found at Harvard Health Publishing at https://www.health.harvard.edu/mind-and-mood/what-is-cognitive-reserve#:~:text=You%20can%20think%20of%20cognitive,lifetime%20of%20education%20and%20curiosity.

25 - Al-Anon Family Group. www.al-anon.org

26 - Langan, Robert C., and Goodbred, Andrew J. Vitamin B12 Deficiency: Recognition and Management. American Family Physician. September 15, 2017. Vol. 96, No. 6, pp. 384-389.

27 - See: https://my.clevelandclinic.org/health/diseases/22831-vitamin-b12-deficiency

28 - According to the National Institute of Health's National Heart, Lung and Blood Institute, pernicious anemia is a condition in which the body cannot make enough healthy red blood cells because it doesn't have enough vitamin B12. The body needs this nutrient to make healthy red blood cells and to keep its nervous system working properly. People who have pernicious anemia cannot absorb enough vitamin B12 from food. This is because they lack intrinsic factor, a protein made in the stomach. A lack of this protein leads to vitamin B12 deficiency. Other conditions and factors also can cause vitamin B12 deficiency. Examples include infections, surgery, medicines, and diet. Technically, the term "pernicious anemia" refers to vitamin B12 deficiency due to a lack of intrinsic factor. Often though, vitamin B12 deficiency due to other causes also is called pernicious anemia. People who suffer from alcoholism may be at risk for pernicious anemia. https://www.nhlbi.nih.gov/health-topics/pernicious-anemia

29 - https://www.webmd.com/drugs/2/drug-77936/namenda-oral/details

30 - https://www.alzheimers.org.uk/about-dementia/types-dementia/korsakoffs-syndrome

31 - https://www.caregiver.org/wernicke-korsakoff-syndrome

32 - https://rarediseases.org/rare-diseases/wernicke-korsakoff-syndrome/

33 - Mace, Nancy L. and Rabins, Peter V. The 36-Hour Day: A Family Guide to Carin for People Who Have Alzheimer Disease, Other Dementia, and Memory Loss. Baltimore, MD. Johns Hopkins University Press. 6th Edition. 2017.

34 - Beller, Jerry. 2020 Wernicke-Korsakoff Syndrome. Heller Health Research Institute, January 2022.

35 - Leatherdale, Lyndsey. Korsakoff's or WKS Explained. Is it Alcohol Induced Dementia. IMB Publishing. 2013.

36 - Clayton and Ninan, Prim Care Companion J Clin Psychiatry. 2010; 12(1): PCC.08r00747. doi: 10.4088/PCC.08r00747blu: 10.4088/PCC.08r00747blu https://www.ncbi.nlm.nih.gov/pmc/articles/PMC2882813/? report=printable 1/21

37 - Conde DM, Verdade RC, Valadares ALR, Mella LFB, Pedro AO, Costa-Paiva L. Menopause and cognitive impairment: A narrative review of current knowledge.

World J Psychiatr 2021; 11(8): 412-428. URL: https://www.wjgnet.com/2220-3206/full/v11/i8/412.htm and DOI: https://dx.doi.org/ 10.5498/wjp.v11.i8.412

38 - O. S. Madueke-Laveaux et al, What We Know about the Long-Term Risks of Hysterectomy for Benign Indication—A Systematic Review, Journal of Clinical Medicine, 2021, volume 10, number 22, 5335. https://doi.org/10. 3390/jcm10225335

39 - See Mayo Clinic, Oophorectomy (ovary removal surgery) at: https://www.mayoclinic.org/tests-procedures/oophorectomy/about/pac-20385030.

40 - Salamon, Maureen, Dementia Link to Early Menopause, Harvard Women's Health Watch, June 1, 2022,
https://www.health.harvard.edu/womens-health/dementia-link-to-early-menopause

41 - D. M. Conde et al, Menopause and cognitive impairment: A narrative review of current Knowledge, World Journal of Psychiatry 2021 August 19, vol 11, number 8, pages 412-428. DOI: 10.5498/wjp.v11.i8.412

42 - Alzheimer's Society, General anaesthetics and dementia. Undated. Downloaded April 2023 at https://www.alzheimers.org.uk/about-dementia/risk-factors-and-prevention/general-anaesthetics

43 - Kushner, Harold S. When Bad Things Happen to Good People. New York, NY. Schocken Books. 1981.

44 - According to Wikipedia, the Serenity Prayer was written by Reinhold Niebuhr, an American theologian. The prayer is normally quoted as: God grant me the serenity to accept things I cannot change, courage to change the things I can, and wisdom to know the difference.

45 - A good initial look at the physiology of dementia can be found in Chapter 3, Characteristic Behavioral Symptoms in People Who Have Dementia, in Nancy L. Mace and Peter Rabins, The 36-Hour Day, Johns Hopkins University Press, Baltimore, 6th Edition, 2017. Also, the Alzheimer's Association has some good visual tutorials on brain physiology at www.alz.org.

46 - https://www.alz.org/alzheimers-dementia/what-is-dementia/types-of-dementia/korsakoff-syndrome

47 - I learned there were two types of exhalation fittings for these ignition-unlock devices. One was the traditional tube which the driver would blow into, and the second style looked like a cup of coffee to-go with the blow-tube hidden from sight. If your loved one accepts or is required to use a breathalyzer, they may find the coffee-cup version more palatable.

48 - Gail Weatherill's book also underscores this point.

49 - The one-time entrance fees for CCRC's are hefty, though the amount varies from CCRC to another. These entrance fees often depend upon several factors, including: 1) the specific size, features and location of the unit desired; 2) whether entering as one or as a couple; 3) the amount of refund that is built into the agreement which would pass along to an heir; 4) the amenities built into the infrastructure and services; and 5) the number of days residents are entitled to live in a nursing care unit.

50 - For more information about CCRCs, a good place to start is the American Association of Retired People (AARP): https://www.aarp.org/caregiving/basics/info-2017/continuing-care-retirement-communities.html

51 - Some CCRCs operate with an alternative model. They charge a higher monthly fee that also increases with each subsequent level of living, versus the financial model I described for our CCRC which requires a large upfront charge but then maintains a relative stable monthly fee regardless of room category (that is, independent, assisted living, memory care, and skilled nursing).

52 - The reader will recall that patients with Korsakoff's Syndrome are not only unaware of their situation, but they are also defensive when others articulate their actual situation.

53 - Readers may recall, Dr. Edwards told us during her review of Nancy's second neuropsychological and her neurological evaluation that another set of evaluations were unnecessary unless circumstances changed.

54 - In the second assessment, she was on the cusp of vulnerability to Alzheimer's Disease and other forms of dementia. Now she was in danger.

55 - Grisel, Judith. Never Enough: The Neuroscience and Experience of Addiction. London, UK. Scribe Publications, 2019.

56 - Kubler-Ross, Elizabeth. On Death and Dying. Scribner Book Company. 50th Anniversary Edition. 2014.

57 - van der Kolk, Bessel. The Body Keeps the Score: Brain, Mind, and Body in the Healing of Trauma. New York, NY. Penguin Books. 2015

58 - Shapiro, Francine. Getting Past Your Past: Take Control of Your Life with Self-Help Techniques from EMDR Therapy. Rodale Press. 2012.

59 - Rasmussen, Christina. Second Firsts: A Step-by-Step Guide to Life after Loss. Carlsbad, CA. Hay House, Inc. 2019.

60 - Rasmussen, Christina. Second Firsts: A Step-by-Step Guide to Life after Loss. Carlsbad, CA. Hay House, Inc. 2019, pp 31-32.

61 - Felten, Eric. Loyalty: The Vexing Virtue. New York. Simon & Shuster Paperbacks. 2011, p. 22.

62 - I am reminded of a memorable line in the 1983 Columbia Pictures movie The Big Chill. Michael Gold (Jeff Goldblum's character) remarked to Sam Weber (played by Tom Berenger) about the need for a few daily rationalizations. See: Wikipedia, The Big Chill, https://en.wikiquote.org/wiki/The_Big_Chill_(film). This film was produced by Michael Shamberg, directed by Lawrence Kasdan, and written by Lawrence Kasdan and Barbara Benedek.

63 - Royce, Josiah. The Philosophy of Loyalty. San Bernardino. Sophia Omni Press. 2017, p 18.

64 - Weatherill, Gail. The Caregiver's Guide to Dementia: Practical Advice for Caring for Yourself and Your Loved One. Emeryville, CA. Rockridge Press. 2020. (Note: readers will also find other self-help books, too, which are focused on dementia caregiving.)

65 - Steele, David J. Blackout: A Look Inside Wernickes. Self-published. 2011. (ISBN: 978-1=105-04395-6).

66 - In Judith Grisel's 2019 book, Never Enough: The Neuroscience and Experience with Addiction, she states that alcohol, while its chemistry is simple, affects more nervous system receptors than opiates and other addictive substances. Therefore, finding a single pharmaceutical medicine that could affect brain chemistry to reduce such craving is a significant challenge.

67 - Butters, N. and Cermak, L.S., Alcoholic Korsakoff's Syndrome. Academic Press, New York. 1980, p. 144.

68 - Rasmussen, Christina. Second Firsts: A Step-by-Step Guide to Life After Loss. Carlsbad, CA. Hay House, Inc. 2019, pp. 103.

# Bibliography and Resources

## Books

Beller, Jerry. *2020 Wernicke Korsakoff Syndrome*. Jerry Heller Health Research Institute. 2019.

Egan, Kerry. *On Living*. New York, NY. Riverhead Books. 2016.

Greitens, Eric. *Resilience: Hard-Won Wisdom for Living a Better Life*. Boston, MA. Mariner Books, Houghton Mifflin Harcourt. 2016.

Grisel, Judith. *Never Enough: The Neuroscience and Experience of Addiction*. London, UK. Scribe Publications. 2019.

Harrison, Thomas F. and Forester, Brent P. *The Complete Family Guide to Dementia*. New York, NY. Guilford Press. 2022.

Kushner, Harold S. *When Bad Things Happen to Good People*. New York, NY. Schocken Books. 1981.

Leatherdale, Lyndsey. *Korsakoff's or Wernicke Korsakoff Syndrome Explained. Is it Alcohol Induced Dementia*. IMB Publishing. 2013.

Mace, Nancy L. and Rabins, Peter V. *The 36-Hour Day: A Family Guide to Caring for People Who Have Alzheimer Disease, Other Dementia, and Memory Loss*. Baltimore, MD. Johns Hopkins University Press. 6th Edition. 2017.

Rasmussen, Christina. *Second Firsts: A Step-by-Step Guide to Life After Loss*. Carlsbad, CA. Hay House, Inc. 2019.

Royce, Josiah. *The Philosophy of Loyalty*. San Bernardino, CA. Sophia Omni Press. 2017.

van der Kolk, Bessel. *The Body Keeps the Score: Brain, Mind, and Body in the Healing of Trauma*. New York, NY. Penguin Books. 2015.

Shapiro, Francine. *Getting Past Your Past: Take Control of Your Life with Self-Help Techniques from EMDR Therapy*. Rodale Press. 2012.

Steele, David J. *Blackout: A Look Inside Wernickes.* Self-published. 2011. ISBN: 978-1-105-04395-6.

Weatherill, Gail. *The Caregiver's Guide to Dementia: Practical Advice for Caring for Yourself and Your Loved One.* Emeryville, CA. Rockridge Press. 2020.

## Organizations

Alzheimer's Association. www.alz.org/alzheimers-dementia/what-is-dementia/types-of-dementia/korsakoff-syndrome

Alzheimer's Society (UK). www.alzheimers.org.uk/about-dementia/types-dementia/korsakoffs-syndrome

Alzheimer's Society, General anaesthetics and dementia. downloaded April 2023 at: https://www.alzheimers.org.uk/about-dementia/risk-factors-and-prevention/general-anaesthetics.

Family Caregiver Alliance. www.caregiver.org/wernicke-korsakoff-syndrome

Hazelden Betty Ford Foundation. www.hazeldenbettyford.org/articles/long-term-alcoholism-can-cause-wet-brain

Cleveland Clinic, Wernicke-Korsakoff's Syndrome. https://my.clevelandclinic.org/health/diseases/22687-wernicke-korsakoff-syndrome

Mountain Springs Recovery. www.mountainspringsrecovery.com

National Institute of Neurological Disorders and Stroke. www.ninds.nih.gov/health-information/disorders/wernick-korsakoff-syndrome

National Organization for Rare Disorders. www.rarediseases.org/rare-diseases/wernicke-korsakoff-syndrome/

WebMD. www.webmd.com/drugs/2/drug-777936/namenda-oral/details

## Selected Scientific and Medical References

The following list of articles and references is by no means comprehensive and is not meant to be a formal review of scientific and medical literature. These references provide the reader with a glimpse of more recent medical findings relevant to Wernicke-Korsakoff Syndrome.


Arts, N.J.M., Walvoort, S.J.W., Kessels, R.P.C. "Korsakoff's Syndrome: a critical review." *Neuropsychiatric Disease and Treatment.* 27. November 2017. Volume 2017: pp. 2875-2890. DOI: https://doi.org/10.2147/NDT.S130078

Billici, R. *et al.* "A case of Wernicke-Korsakoff Syndrome treated one year after the onset of symptoms." *Primary Care Companion for CNS Disorders.* 2015; 17(6):10.4008/PCC.15/01801. https://www.psychiatrist.com/PCC/article/Pages/2015/v17n06/15101801.aspx

Birnbaum, I.M. and Parker, E.S, editors. *Alcohol and Human Memory.* Routledge, London, and New York. 2017. [originally published by Lawrence Erlbaum Associates, Hillsdale, NJ, 1977.]

Butters, Nelson and Cermak, Laird. *Alcoholic Korsakoff's Syndrome: An Information-Processing Approach to Amnesia.* Academic Press. New York. 1980.

Chandra Kumar, A., Bhardwaj, A., and W. 't Jong, G. "Review of thiamine disorders, Wernicke encephalopathy and Korsakoff psychosis." *Journal of Basic Clinical Pharmacology*, 2019, Vo. 30, No. 2, pp. 153-162. https://pubmed.ncbi.nlm.nih.gov/30281514/

Clayton and Ninan, "Depression or Menopause: Presentation and Management of Major Depressive Disorder in Perimenopausal and Post menopausal Women." *Prim Care Companion J Clin Psychiatry*, 2010; 12(1): PCC.08r00747. DOI: 10.4088/PCC.08r00747blu: 10.4088/PCC.08r00747blu and https://www.ncbi.nlm.nih.gov/pmc/articles/PMC2882813/?report=printable 1/21

Conde D.M., Verdade R.C., Valadares A.L.R., Mella L.F.B., Pedro A.O., Costa-Paiva L. "Menopause and cognitive impairment: A narrative review of current knowledge." *World Journal of Psychiatry.* 2021. Vol. 11, issue 8, pages 412-428. https://www.wjgnet.com/2220-3206/full/v11/i8/412.htm, and DOI: https://dx.doi.org/10.5498/wjp.v11.i8.412

Covell, Timothy and Siddiqui, Waquar. *Korsakoff Syndrome.* StatPearls Publishing LLC. January 2023. https://www.ncbi.nlm.nih.gov/books/NBK539854/

Langan, Robert C., and Goodbred, Andrew J. "Vitamin B12 Deficiency: Recognition and Management." *American Family Physician.* September 15, 2017. Vol. 96, No. 6, pp. 384-389. https://pubmed.ncbi.nlm.nih.gov/28925645/

Madueke-Laveaux, O.S., *et al.* "What We Know about the Long-Term Risks of Hysterectomy for Benign Indication—A Systematic Review." *Journal of Clinical Medicine.* 2021. Vol. 10, number 22, 5335. https://doi.org/10.3390/jcm10225335

Mayo Clinic, Oophorectomy (ovary removal surgery) at https://www.mayoclinic.org/tests-procedures/oophorectomy/about/pac-20385030

Richter, Derek, ed. *Addiction and Brain Damage.* Routledge. London and New York. 2017. [originally published by Croom Helm, Ltd. London. 1980.]

Ross, Julie D., Gastfriend, David R., and Renner Jr, John A. "Chapter 14 - Alcoholic Patients: Acute and Chronic." *Massachusetts General Hospital Handbook of General Hospital Psychiatry* (Sixth Edition). 2010. pp. 153-162.

Salamon, M. "Dementia Link to Early Menopause." *Harvard Women's Health Watch.* June 1, 2022. https://www.health.harvard.edu/womens-health/dementia-link-to-early-menopause

Sanvisens, Arantza *et al.* "Long-term mortality of patients with an alcohol-related Wernicke-Korsakoff Syndrome." *Alcohol and Alcoholism.* Vol.

52, Issue 4, July 2017. pp. 466-471. www.academic.oup.com/alcalc/article/52/4/4661/3065162

Smith, I. and Hillman, A. "Management of alcohol Korsakoff Syndrome." *Advances in Psychiatric Treatment*. 1999. Vol. 5, pp. 271-278. https://www.researchgate.net/publication/255608445_Management_of_Alcohol_Korsakoff_Syndrome

Thomson, A.D., Guerrini, I, and Marshall, E.J. "The Evolution and Treatment of Korsakoff's Syndrome: Out of Sight, Out of Mind?" *Neuropsychology Review*. June 2012:22(2): 81-92. https://doi.org/10.1007/s11065-012-9196-z

Thomson, A.D., and Marshall, E.J. "The natural history and pathophysiology of Wernicke's encephalopathy and Korsakoff's psychosis." *Alcohol and Alcoholism*. 2006. Vol. 41. Pp.151-158. https://doi.org/10.1093/alcalc/agh249

van Dam, M.J., van Meijel, B., Postma, A., Oudman, E. "Health problems and care needs in patients with Korsakoff's Syndrome: A systematic review." *Journal of Psychiatric and Mental Health Nursing*. 2020. Vol. 27, pp.460-481. https://research.vumc.nl/en/publications/health-problems-and-care-needs-in-patients-with-korsakoffs-syndro

## Also, see Science Direct and Google Scholar for more resources:

https://www.sciencedirect.com/topics/medicine-and-dentistry/korsakoff-psychosis

https://scholar.google.com/scholar?hl=en&as_sdt=0%2C5&q=wernicke+korsakoff+syndrome&oq=wernic

# About Atmosphere Press

Founded in 2015, Atmosphere Press was built on the principles of Honesty, Transparency, Professionalism, Kindness, and Making Your Book Awesome. As an ethical and author-friendly hybrid press, we stay true to that founding mission today.

If you're a reader, enter our giveaway for a free book here:

SCAN TO ENTER
BOOK GIVEAWAY

If you're a writer, submit your manuscript for consideration here:

SCAN TO SUBMIT
MANUSCRIPT

And always feel free to visit Atmosphere Press and our authors online at atmospherepress.com. See you there soon!

# About the Author

**Karl Muller** has over 40 years of experience in science, technology, and health risk communications from his work in both public and private sector organizations. He graduated with a master's degree from a major university in the US. Karl has lived and worked in the United States and abroad.

*The author may be contacted at karlmullerthebook@gmail.com.*